DANCING ON THE VERGE OF DAWN

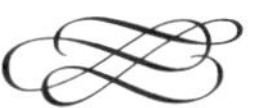

DANCING ON THE VERGE OF DAWN

FINDING HOPE IN DARK STORMS AND MOMENTS ALONE -
AN ANTHOLOGY OF STORIES BY WOMEN OF FAITH
WRITTEN DURING THE PANDEMIC OF 2020

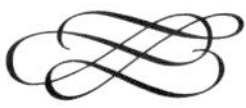

ELLEN JANZEN

with

ELLA H., HOPE HESSED, MICHELLE H., WENDY
KONEMANN, SHARON MACDONALD, NADIA M.,
ROBYN NEUFELD, MICHELLE P., AIMEE ROOF, SARAH
BAHIRAEI, NANCY WILLIAMS, LOUISE C. WOOD

MOF PUBLISHING

Paperback: 978-0-9958951-5-7

Ebook: 978-0-9958951-6-4

Cover painting by Serena S.

Layout and formatting by MOF Publishing.

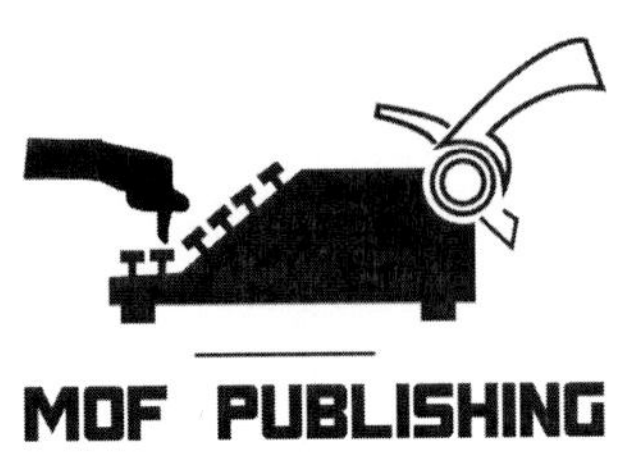

To all those who embrace the dance.

CONTENTS

CONTRIBUTORS

Contributions to this book were made by these friends:

Nancy Williams is a Licensed Marriage and Family Therapist, a perinatal educator and consultant. She taught at a university at both the undergrad and graduate levels, specializing in Human Development. She is a Disaster Relief Chaplain for the Southern Baptists, as well as a consultant/trainer with Care Net (pregnancy center ministries). As the mother of three children, a grandmother to nine, a great-grandmother to two, the wife of a pastor and a sister to a cross-cultural worker, she has gleaned more than her fair share of experience and insight. She has co-authored a great book on human connection, *The Stone Age Baby in a Techno Society*.

Sarah Vosseteig Bahiraei is a Midwesterner (from the USA) who hopped on a plane to Turkey in 2014 with a one-way ticket in hand. She lives there with her husband, where they work in refugee ministry. They are expecting their first child in 2020. She writes about her faith, immigration and living the in-between on her blog onefootonboth.com.

Robyn Neufeld is an Australian, currently residing in Sydney, whose life outside her native land for more than half her life, primarily in the Middle East, greatly impacted her life and values. She is passionate about Jesus, and loves partnering with Him to see people walk in joy, health and freedom. She has been married to her soulmate, Matt, for more than 30 years. They share four amazing children (one in heaven), a son-in-law, and two gorgeous grandchildren. She is a relational coach and counsellor.

Wendy Konemann, a trained counsellor, is heavily involved in biblical peace-making as a writer, speaker, trainer, conflict coach and mediator. Recommending her on so many levels, she has walked 1000 kilometres on *El Camino* (The Way) twice. She is passionate about connecting people to God in the midst of their struggles.

Ella H. prefers to go anonymously into these pages; she is a woman gifted with insight and grace. And that is enough.

Louise C. Wood has lived most of her adult life outside of her birth / passport country. That journey has not been straight forward and she has moved several times— sometimes abruptly. She is deeply encouraged by seeing how the Lord weaves her story into a beautiful whole.

Aimee Roof, following her namesake, is first the beloved and friend. She spent five of the last 10 years living abroad, is a life-long learner, one who loves to sit at Jesus' feet and loves to guide other women in finding wholeness and healing as an Integrative Nutrition Health Coach. BeWholeHealthCoaching.wordpress.com

Nadia M., as a young single woman, has lived cross culturally for over three years. Her passion—to bring the love of God to those she meets and her commitment to find God's presence in her daily life—qualifies her to speak into the lives of those who read her story or walk by her side.

Sharon MacDonald has multiple layers of experience of working with people in the "outsider" category—from Alzheimer residents, brain injured people, stroke victims, to just ordinary cross-cultural relationships. She also translates regularly for the deaf. All this set her up for 10 years as a flight attendant where she had opportunities to see the world and give service to anyone she met along the way, but most fulfilling were the days she combined her love for special needs with the "ordinary" job.

Michelle P. has lived and breathed the sandy air of West Africa for nearly twenty years. She and her partner, equally persistent by nature, work in development projects while raising a vibrant family of five.

Michelle H. met Mark at college. After hearing him sing, "People need the Lord," in a chapel service, they became best friends, sharing a vision to live cross-cultur-ally. They were married, and after a few years of searching to discover their specific calling, they moved to North Africa in 1996. There, Michelle served as an English teacher for the first two years, and then as a wife and mom, active in the local church. After their youngest child was diagnosed with autism in 2005, they moved into ministry with local families facing the same challenge. Mark was particularly motivated to reach fathers in order to help them connect with and nurture their families. In 2019 Mark died under tragic circumstances that left Michelle and her autistic son traumatized and in need of professional care for healing. They moved to the United States, to the town where her daughter and son-in-law, Anita and Tim, live.

Hope Hessed has spent 40 (of her 60) years as a single woman. Hope dealt with the significant isolation this brings. She lives in a rural North African culture where she struggles to learn how to be an alien from a privileged minority.

Ellen Janzen is a mom, a granny, a writer, a gardener and a sojourner. Ellen does family coaching and bilingualism education, sometimes combining both. She also provides spiritual journey companionship. She has written a couple of books that you can find on Amazon—*The Day the Mountains Crashed into the Sea* and *The Unspoken Gospel*—reflecting her passion for gifts of wisdom that come wrapped in a good story. You can find out more at ellenjanzen.com.

"Serena" did the artwork for the cover, which tells its own story!

Kathleen Ibsen gave insight and editorial advice to the content of this book and helped in the journey toward discovering a good title. She is a writer, a chaplain, a spiritual director, and an exceptional friend.

The writers of this book are from five countries. The grammar, spelling and punctuation of each chapter reflects the rules and preferences used in those various country of origin. Believe it or not, Canada, the USA, Britain and Australia all have their own preferences for punctuation. Feel free to spot which writer is from your country if you are a native English speaker. Two of the contributors are not native English speakers—their work has been edited by a Canadian.

WELCOME TO THE DANCE OF LIFE

Somewhere, inside each of us, there is the capacity to step into the rhythm of relationship with others: the rhythm of connections that give our lives meaning. Including, of course, the relationship we have with our Creator. We were made for the rhythm of connection. In that dance we observe—

• it is a dance that is most often un-choreographed, unrepeatable;

• we don't know what will happen next until we are in the "turn" or twirl that takes us to the next sequence of moves;

• it is a dance that is rarely without mistakes—they add to the excitement and adventure, as life was meant to be an adventure;

• it can be very tiring, our feet grow weary and stiff, but we dance on;

• it is a dance where one takes the lead and another follows—but make no mistake, someone is the leader.

We dedicate this book to all of you who read it.
May you find the grace to keep on dancing
when you find yourself in the rain on a dark night
when you find yourself dangerously close to a storm
when you find yourself alone…

Know this: the One who loves you most,
knows the rhythm of this dance.
Let your feet follow His
and you will never be lost.

INTRODUCTION

Welcome to our book of true tales—A book of perhaps wildly different stories with accompanying thoughts and reflections.

Some stories are strange, a little unbelievable. Others are filled with wonder—awe at what God has done. Some are strange with wonder—some of us have lived adventurous lives that sound exotic. Or, you might say, the journeys we have followed have been full of challenge.

And some are stories that are as close to normal as you can get…yet no one leads an ordinary life. We are all equally connected to the eternal God who made us—extraordinary. Extra ordinary.

The writers, from five different countries, span in age from their 20s to their 80s. Joined to each other by friendship—most are my (Ellen's) friends. And through the themes explored in this book we are pieced together like a stained-glass window, each of us holding the light in a different hue.

"In true community we are windows constantly offering each other new views on the mystery of God's presence in our lives."[1]

We all need windows—sunshine and fresh air are essential to our health.

Windows open our lives up to the world outside, in this case, the outside world sees into our inner spaces.

This book of windows is like a poster of doors you sometimes find when you travel. Some doors in the poster are brightly painted, others are old and weathered. Some are wide and others are small.

While the windows in this book are deliberately "mis-matched" they carry one theme. I invited my friends to write about experiences that prepared them for the COVID-19 crisis of social distancing, isolation…quarantine. Each chapter is written to draw us in to participate in this journey of discovery. Between the chapters are placed "Interludes" that are reflections on the themes of journeying with God.

Some of us chose to share stories that tie us to the current situation of facing the current changes in social context, the challenges of living with COVID-19 restrictions. Some are less obviously written for the reason of answering the question raised during this pandemic.

What question? Have we asked the question? Or questions?

The question is this: How are you coping in the shifting and restricting world crisis that has unravelled our communities and pushed us toward isolation? Are you managing? Are you just barely coping?

Or are you finding yourself digging deeper into the faith that God is present to us and with us in this difficulty? A God who specializes in showing up in the hardest of times—even when…especially when we have a hard time feeling or noticing his nearness.

David, in the Psalms, cries out to God with his question during a time that I assume, defies the feeling of God's presence with him. He asks over and over, "How long, O Lord? How long will you forget me?"[2]

Sometimes the process of discovery is a long and painful one. It seems that quite often, hopelessness precedes seeking and seeking precedes discovery. But the good news is that discovery is never just the "same old, same old." Discovery is, by nature, that there is something new ahead. Something fresh and delightful…and good.

It is our hope—the hope of each person who contributed to this book of "windows"—that you will find that there is a secret agenda in this hard time. That the purposes of God are for you to discover His love and presence in a different, deeper, more fulfilling way during this challenging time. And this is a timeless message—it will still be true long after the masks are put away and COVID-19 is a fading memory.

We hope our windows light your way—that through the lens of our writing you will be inspired to look again.

Where is God showing up for you in this time? How is He leading you into His presence with the rhythms of grace—hope and love and truth when times are hardest? How are you learning to lean in and dance with Him, following the pattern of His presence?

We hope our stories inspire confidence that God is meeting you at every turn. And the more you get connected, the easier it is for God to take the lead.

---

1. Henri Nouwen, "Making all things new," in *The Spiritual Life: Eight Essential Titles*, New York, Harper Collins, 2016.
2. Psalm 13:1.

DEEP, DEEP LOVE

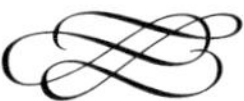

NANCY WILLIAMS

Lockdown. Quarantine. Isolation. Social distance.

As I write, we are well into the second month of mandatory aloneness. We are designed by God, the Trinity Who is the ultimate community, to live with and among others. We are created to be bonded to those around us. Our biological expectation drives us to attachment.

Yet here we are.

During our Easter isolation, I pondered what Saturday must have been like for Jesus' followers, after the crucifixion. Though Jesus had told them all what would happen, they did not understand.

It's Saturday. The Day After. The horror of that terrible Friday is over. There is calm. Sabbath Rest. And prohibition for those who loved Him, longing to tend to His body. And He is gone. Expected deliverance unfulfilled.

Disappointment, grief, devastation.

While we probably can't understand the seriousness and intensity of what His followers were facing, we have all experienced Saturday. Darkness, hopelessness, fear of the unknown. Many people are now feeling the helplessness of a forced rest when we want to be tending to something.

Isolated forced rest. Unaccompanied in grief. On our own in the grip of fear.

While most of us have never faced anything like a pandemic prior to current events, we most likely have experienced something like the loneliness that many of us are experiencing. So many circumstances brought by life have similar feelings.

Physical pain is isolating. People can try and help, be supportive, bring food, pray for us and yet no one can help me bear the pain. The best example of this is a laboring woman working to bring her child into the world. She may have a very loving supportive husband. She might have hired a caring doula. Good midwives or nurses may compassionately attend to her. Yet she is the only one feeling the pain of her contractions. Yes, a body of research tells us that because of neurochemical release, the presence of these empathetic people in the room will actually alleviate the discomfort and allow the mother to progress towards birth much more efficiently.

Emotional pain isn't much different except that it is harder to qualify. We need people to be with us. I would imagine that on that terrible Sabbath Saturday that His followers sought the company of others. Maybe limited to those under their roof but in this collective society people would unquestionably seek the comfort of their familiar human attachments. I often wonder if Westerners have simply lost the instinct to shelter in the loving shadow of others.

As a therapist, I have seen that during prolonged isolation there are more suicide attempts and self-harm, seriously increased anxiety and depression, severely exacerbated domestic violence and the deafening sounds of the silence of loneliness for the elderly and infirm.

Many of us are spared the intensity of that depth of suffering. Yes, everyone struggles. Each of us has our own valley to walk through during various points of our lives. It can be common to have our "emotional circuits" shut down or shorting out. Our relationships with God and others somehow go awry and we find ourselves trying to cope, to compensate in unhealthy ways. For some, this means extra trips to the refrigerator. Others may find themselves "checking out" by spending hours playing on the computer or reading. Still more may find themselves using substances or other addictions as a substitute for relationship. The very behaviors that offer us momentary relief prove, in the end, to create more isolation and more pain.

Our current Saturday experience is made that much worse by the fact that there are no coaches or doulas in the room with us. And yet…… Emmanuel sits as the God who is with us, just waiting for us to turn and acknowledge Him.

Aloneness is not the state that we were designed for. Thinking that we can ignore our need for others, for connection with God is to thumb our nose at His very creation. If loneliness is the poison, perhaps we would consider the God-given antidote.

Alcoholics Anonymous has a saying, "You are only as sick as your secrets." So often, rather than reaching out, we find ourselves hiding out in our secret emotional caves.

There was a time earlier in my life when I was in terrible emotional pain, walking through the most serious crisis of my life. The worst of it was that I feared that God had abandoned me in my questions and suffering. Of course, I prayed, but did not have any assurance that He was listening, caring, or acting. My mind was dark with fear and my heart hard with mistrust. And then one afternoon while my kids were napping and I was doing laundry, I had a cassette tape playing, *"Oh the Deep, Deep Love of Jesus."*

Strangely enough—or perhaps not strange at all—while I was doing the most mundane of tasks, folding underwear, everything changed. Suddenly I was wrapped in a blanket of His comforting presence. It felt as though I was being rocked in a chair like a crying child. I heard no words, except the words playing in the song. I needed no words. What I needed was the loving touch that He gave me.

Often that is our hearts cry towards God and towards any people around us. "I just need a hug." "Could you just sit and listen?" "Hold my hand as we walk through this."

Emmanuel, this God who is with us, is not sitting across the room. The idea behind this is that He is actually pressed into us from all sides, whatever they may be. And He has given us the Body of Christ to hug us as well.

What a kind, loving God we have!

ABOUT THE AUTHOR

My husband met Nancy at a conference and came home with the report that I would love this woman—whom one day I would meet. I've come to trust him when he says this to me. Nancy is funny and fun and deeply serious. She has become a great friend, a mentor, and one of the most encouraging people in my life. She encourages me not just through her words, but through her whole-hearted service around the world. She has been to more countries, with more teams, investing in more women than anyone else I know. I'm so grateful she joined this story-telling journey that we've invited you to share. I hope one day you meet Nancy or someone just as generous and kind, who believes in you.

INTERLUDE: SONG OF HEAVEN

MICHELLE P.

A song
An anthem of heaven
A song sung from every corner of the skies
The Saints gone before
The creation's echoes
The angels dance
A Song that's far greater than those who sing it
A song of the goodness of the Lord

It swirls around me
It calls me on
It pushes me forward
It lifts me up
A song around me
A song within me
A glory song
A love song
A victory song
A song of mercy
A song of desperation
A song of lament
A song of victory

A song of the goodness of the Lord

It's sung from the highest mountain
It's sung from the widest beach
It's sung in stillness and silence
It's sung in the chaos and noise
It's sung in the darkest crevices of the deepest valleys
It's sung from the hills of celebration
It's sung on the journey of brokenness
It's sung by the rivers of restoration
It's sung in the marketplace of promise
It's sung by the graveyard of goodbyes

My heart beats with this song.
I am caught up in the glory
I am part of something far bigger than I am
My voice, my heart, my soul beating with the song
In every season
A song of the goodness of the Lord

LITTLE JOY CRUMBS

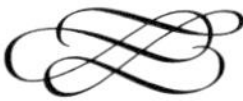

SARAH BAHIRAEI

A tiny foot is wedged into the bottom of my ribcage, prompting me to surrender to third-trimester insomnia and rise with the spring sun. I make coffee, pulling down the same two mugs I always do for my husband and myself. It is a daily rhythm serving as an anchor in these strange times where one day bleeds into the next.

Today the coffee brews over the gas stovetop because of a neighborhood power outage—a small inconvenience, but I have lived abroad long enough to expect interruptions. It comes with the package when signing up for the expatriate life.

But how troubling it is the first time the veil of certainty is stolen from our startled hands and we realize we were not as in control as we once thought. How troubling it is when a novel virus carries itself invisibly from street to street, city to city, and we all find ourselves behind the closed doors of our homes, our routines wholly and completely upset. "Normal" holds a new definition now, the old meaning tossed aside. One day it was and the next it was not.

My husband and I have had good practice braving the onset of life's interruptions. Prolonged uncertainty breeds isolation but we have learned to receive it. Along with living in a foreign country, we got married amid a controversial travel ban, paddled the choppy waters of immigration visas, and are now bringing a child into a worldwide pandemic. Uncertainty is an always-present third party perched on top of the couch, a visitor who has missed the cues and overstayed its welcome.

Like brewing coffee, walking outside each day—perhaps more of a waddle, belly propelling me forward—has been another anchor, a sacred cadence for the soul.

Neighboring homes stand stoic and taciturn as families tuck themselves inside. The unusual silence cloaks everything like a stubborn layer of dust. There are masked faces, parks wrapped in police tape, canceled plans, and disappointments.

But when looking a little more closely, there is also a wave of a hand from a watchful grandma behind glass, a clumsily colored rainbow taped to a window, a softer and gentler greeting between two people as they pass six feet apart. A turtle ambles across the rocks. The lilac trees blossom into soft purples. A collared dove perched in an evergreen calls out in a long, slow lament.

Having weathered many upsets in life, my husband and I know the feeling of juggling juxtaposing emotions. At the beginning of the year, we received news that caused the seams of our life to unravel and the ground beneath our feet to shake. The heartbeat of every one of our prayers for the last few years was for a single door to open. And now, after one phone call with an impassive immigration clerk on the other end of the line, that door was closed shut.

Yet life went on and my belly grew a little rounder each day. A week after receiving the devastating news, we held a party with our close friends where we bit into cupcakes to the count of three and cheered when little pink sprinkles spilled out from the middle—a girl. We celebrated with frosting decorating the corners of our laughing mouths, sprinkles falling into cupped hands. And I remember feeling these words dash across my mind for just a fleeting moment: This is kind of nice.

When receiving the difficult news earlier that week, all our future dreams dissipated in front of us. We could no longer plan ahead. The curtain of certainty was stolen and replaced with an unending today but never tomorrow. But this—celebrating the coming of a new baby girl with pink cupcakes and laughs and prayers —was nice.

The late poet, Mary Oliver, writes that joy should not be compared to a crumb. Recognizing the scattering of little joy crumbs on the counters of our lives does not need to be embarrassingly brushed into our hands and down the sink or quickly wiped from our lips before anyone has noticed. "If you suddenly and unexpectedly feel joy," she pens, "don't hesitate. Give in to it." We have permission to recognize the little bit of beauty in the struggles of life.

Spotting joy—there it is and there is another!—does not overshadow the weight of grief, disappointment, and pain, for these too, are important to hold. Feeling one thing does not negate the other because both/and fits comfortably on our laps.

Joy makes space for these heavy things. We can lift it onto one hip and sorrow the other, our arms wrapped around both like a mother gathering her children to her. It is in the tension of life's complications where the scent of God is. It is here—right here, at this moment—where the Creator speaks, for he holds it all together. At this crossroads is where we can partake in the glory that will be revealed at God's coming again.

Joy is in the kick of a tiny baby's foot, the slow brew of morning coffee, a power outage, the daily rhythm of rising and opening curtains. It is in a leisurely walk, the still small whisper of God's voice, two mugs set out on the table, frosting on a cupcake. Perhaps looking for these is a way to fight back against the heaviness of life. Perhaps it is okay to see a morsel of joy in the middle of pain.

So, when you do see little joy crumbs do not hesitate. Give in to it. Grab on to it.

ABOUT THE AUTHOR

I met Sarah when she attended a workshop I was leading. She didn't say much in the large group. I should have known that there was more beneath the quiet surface! As soon as I started reading her blog, I felt like I had met an old friend. I am amazed by what she knows in her first decade of adulthood. I was not nearly so wise in my youth. Sarah's writing is sprinkled throughout the book; do visit her blog—it's worth the trip! onefootonboth.com

INTERLUDE: THE SMELL OF FRESH RAIN

ELLEN JANZEN

When a baby arrives in the world, all five senses are calibrated as a connection indicator, seeking closeness to their caregiver (usually mother). This connection is essential to survival. The design of this dance between parent and child is a stunning expression of how intricately we are "knit together."

Each of our five senses activates one or more of our body's regulatory features—how we breathe, our heart rate, temperature, digestion and more.

Even the connection itself is an intricate exchange with one partner taking the lead —initiating contact—and the other following with a response. This dance builds trust that leads to a lifetime's ability to enter relationships with healthy emotions and expectations.

The baby's initial connection to caregiver develops the limbic and cognitive centres in the brain, giving an infant a place to find tranquility. When children feel safe in the arms of their parents, they flourish both physically and emotionally. Our five senses are designed to highlight awareness of safety and place us into a calm state where growth is optimal.

Sadly, many of us have experiences in our early childhood that are lodged in our limbic memory—times we were anxious and not protected, threatened and not cared for, or frustrated and not acknowledged. That dance was combative rather than comforting.

Our inner "normal" created by our emotional history is not one that is calm and restful for our own thoughts and feelings. Some of us live with a heightened awareness of our "fight or flight warning" on a low setting—but still warning mode, on all the time. We are easily thrown into a flashing red light "RUN" warning.

One of the gifts that we can turn to in times of anxiety and futility is the gift of our physical senses. When we see something soothing (leaves rustling in the wind, fire licking at darkness), we can focus and allow a calm inner space to form inside us—physically and emotionally. The sound of the sea, or of rain on the roof—these invite us to grow quiet in our inner space. When we sit in a bath of warm water, with the scent of lavender floating off the soap, it can be similar to the safety of life before birth—a time when most of us did not experience extreme stress.

If we had a place of safety and tranquility to come "home to" as a child, we can easily find the place of calm when we pause to focus in a still place. At the same time, we can start to create connections of peace even if they were sparse in our childhood.

If you can't find calm easily through the portal of your thoughts, it is not wrong or deficient to pay attention to your body as a source of connection. Slow your breathing, feel the earth beneath your feet, smell the scent of fresh rain (if you can) and engage in the current moment with your five senses.

Sitting outside with a light breeze on my face, listening to the birds and feeling the grass under my bare feet are some of my favourite ways to experience the calming of my inner world through the gift of my five senses. The sound of rain, or ocean waves, or of the wind in the trees also bring me to inner stillness.

If gazing at the sun as it rises, or watching it slowly sink over the horizon, gives you a sense of well-being—brings you to tranquility—that is the gift you can and should invest in. If listening to the sea is your go-to for recalibrating your soul, then go sit by the sea, or go fishing whenever you are able. If you love the forest, go there to walk, take photos and even just touch the bark on a lovely old tree.

If you are truly stuck indoors, there is less potential for some of these—but perhaps with creativity you can find a few ways to connect through your five senses—sitting at an open window or lingering on a rooftop terrace. Get a set of paints and feel the brush as it runs colour over a canvas—choose the colour to heighten or express your mood and emotion. If nothing else, listen to a recording on YouTube. The song "All Things Bright and Beautiful" was written in order to awaken children to the wonder of being made in God's image and the gifts of connection to him through the five senses.

Those moments of paying attention to what your senses are telling you are essential to creating a flourishing place in your life.

The awareness of the beauty of the present moment is a gift that God has built into our human bodies—connecting our skin, ears, eyes, and hands to our limbic brain —our emotional centre. It isn't necessarily "spiritual" to breathe slowly and feel your heartbeat slow down. It is part of our design for connection—and it can be very effective in connecting us to the One who created each of us. Peace and hope are part of what is offered when we tune our senses into His presence.

Chances are very good you will find yourself in the presence of a God who waits to protect you and provide for your inner needs. The One who sees you, also sings over you... wraps you in his wings and offers you a feast—the imagery of how God meets you with His expressions of presence through the five senses are generously described throughout the Bible.

Psalm 104:5-7

> *He set the earth on its foundations;*
> *it can never be moved.*
> *You covered it with the watery depths as with a garment;*
> *the waters stood above the mountains.*
> *But at your rebuke the waters fled,*
> *at the sound of your thunder they took to flight;*

Isaiah 25:6

> *On this mountain the Lord Almighty will prepare a feast of rich food for all peoples, a banquet of aged wine — the best of meats and the finest of wines.*

Job 26:9

> *He covers the face of the full moon, spreading his clouds over it.*

Deuteronomy 11:11

> *But the land you are crossing the Jordan to take possession of is a land of mountains and valleys that drinks rain from heaven.*

Song of Songs 4:16

> "Awake, north wind, and come, south wind! Blow on my garden, that its
> fragrance may spread everywhere. Let my beloved come into his garden
> and taste its choice fruits."

Not surprisingly, God expresses himself through the five senses. He delights in us in ways that are not unusual or uncommon—but too often we have not noticed.

Truly, the smell of fresh rain is a divine gift.

THE GIFTS OF SLOWING DOWN

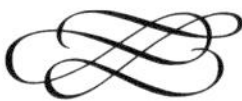

ROBYN NEUFELD

Slowing down. I always had the choice, but somehow I thought it was indulgent.

Just before we went into physical distancing mode (I like to call it that rather than social distancing, as we still need social connection even if it isn't physical) I had coffee with a dear friend, and told her how Matt and I had been planning to have a couple of weeks at our beach house to rest (something we haven't ever done).

We often come here to "work" – clean, garden, prepare for renters or run workshops. We have committed ourselves to a daily walk along the beach whenever we are here. Although we are only 100 km from Sydney, it feels very remote and tranquil. We have an amazing view of the Pacific Ocean in one direction and Brisbane Water, an inlet, in the other. Sunrises and sunsets are stunning: being close to the water feeds my soul.

Our plan to have two weeks here didn't happen due to a sudden family crisis the previous month. I joked with Wendy, "Maybe if we went overseas we would be forced into two weeks isolation on our return." She looked at me quite seriously and said, "You could just choose to rest."

Wise words. Well less than two weeks later we found ourselves at our beach house where we have (mostly) been for the last seven plus weeks. Here I am at the place I wanted to be, where I wanted to rest, forced by my government and a virus that is greatly impacting the world as we have known it.

I know I am incredibly blessed.

I am an extrovert, so I do miss connecting with the people I love. I miss greetings and hugging people. I miss visiting my dad and playing Rummy Cube with him.

But there have been a lot of gifts in this time.

The gift of connection.

Given the nature of my life (living more than half of it outside my native land), I have parts of my heart all over the globe. I've lived in places where uncertainty was the norm for a long time. But this is the first time where everyone in the world is impacted in some way by this new way of living. Connecting with those far away has been precious – siblings, Matt's cousins, precious teammates we partnered with two decades ago, colleagues sharing inspiring stories from their foreign ministry.

The gift of creativity.

Matt has been working on two beautiful mosaic outdoor coffee tabletops that he's been wanting to do for a couple of years. The first one is an adaptation of a famous Japanese woodblock print, *The Great Wave of Kanagawa*. Now infused with the prophetic word of forward momentum, it brings joy and beauty to our terrace. The second one, a lighthouse, has many special meanings for us – Rhode Island, the place of Susanna's birth, is rich in lighthouses, our dear friends, Doug and Patti have named their beach house in Oregon *"El Manar"* (the lighthouse), and other dear friends in Egypt, Ramses and Vinis, have a ministry named "Lighthouse."

I've been working on a photo book of the Camino journey we did two years ago. It's been a precious time of reminiscing and remembering. I've also been practicing classical piano pieces – something I've been meaning to do but haven't got around to. Sometimes when we Skype my dad, I play a piece for him – a special connection.

The gift of nature.

We never tire of the beauty of this place. The bush, the bay and the beach (as the locals boast!). We get to walk in this beautiful environment every day. The beach is not crowded, but we see people walking their dogs. As we pass and greet them (people and dogs) – from an acceptable distance — it's starting to feel familiar.

The beach changes. I didn't know that. I've never spent such an extended time near the beach to see how the sand fills the rock pools, then empties them again. How sand dunes are formed, and then flattened. To see the ocean fierce and majestic one day, and then calm and pacific the next.

To hear the kookaburras calling, see the sparrows darting, and the rosellas bringing their splash of colour to the trees in our yard. And speaking of a splash of colour – the Tibuchina! I didn't even know this plant existed a year ago, until it burst into glorious purple flower last autumn, and bursting again it is now. A native of Central and South America, it has graciously found a home in my garden. A grace indeed.

The gift of connection with God.

This has been a special space for me in this time. As I said, I am an extrovert, so inviting others into my God-space brings me joy. Three young women have asked me to mentor them (remotely), so that's been a life-giving time of being present to God in His word. I have been blessed by some contemplative apps that have helped me to be present to God on a daily basis. We get to attend church (and our fellowship group) online, which we feel very blessed to do.

Matt and I attended an online conference that inspired us and filled us with hope. We are now offering an online workshop in order to pass on our blessing to others. So many ways to give and receive and be present.

The gift of memories. As I mentioned, I've been putting together a photo book of the Camino, which has meant reading through my journal. This memory touched me today:

"We decided to have an early start today – 7am – which was still in the dark. Such a beautiful time of day to be on the way. We saw the sun rise, which was magnificent. When it was still dark, the clouds seemed like one continuous mass, but once the light started filtering through, shape and texture became apparent. I thought about how life can be like that, especially the problems we sometimes face – one seeming mass. Yet when light is allowed to filter through, we notice different layers, textures. It's not just one big mass. And then the light brings beauty and we are able to embrace the new day."

This rang true as I reflected on our experience these last couple of months. Hearing about the virus and the danger seemed like a huge dark mass. We have made sacrifices as we try to stem the ravages we feared. And gradually the light is filtering through and exposing the gifts that are available. May we embrace each day and may our lives post-COVID-19 be richer, slower and more gracious because of our new eyes. Our new experiences. Our new hope.

Slowing down. A choice I'm embracing.

ABOUT THE AUTHOR

Have you ever met someone that you instinctively know you will be friends with? Maybe it was her soft Australian accent and gentle manner or perhaps it was the sparkle in her earrings that gave me that sense—Here is a friend I want to get to know. We've looked forward to enjoying time with each other at international gatherings for almost 20 years now. I don't see Robyn often, but here is what she means to me—when she handed me an invitation to her daughter's wedding, I said "I would love to come." And I did, even though it meant driving 30 hours to the neighbouring country! She means that much to me.

INTERLUDE: WAITING FOR THE SUN TO RISE

SARAH BAHIRAEI

Every night during the month of Ramadan (or Ramazan as it's called in Turkey), our town is awakened by the steady beating of a drum. Dressed in traditional Ottoman attire, the drummer weaves his way up and down the neighborhood streets with a stick in one hand and a drum in the other. A ritual dating back hundreds of years, the drum's purpose is to awaken the locals to begin preparing for *sahur*, the last meal eaten before the sun rises. The neighbors begin to stir and kitchen lights slowly click on, giving off a dull glow behind window shades.

The beating gets softer as the drummer moves on to the next neighborhood. I let the curtain fall back to its place and crawl into bed. The nights are warmer now so we sleep with thin sheets and open windows. The dog next door barks in reply to the sound of the drum. I flip over my phone on the nightstand to check the time. It's 2:30 am.

The other evening, after we had finished washing dishes and cleaning up dinner, my husband and I walked by the river running through our town. Each picnic table was occupied with multi-generational families. Savory smoke swirled out from miniature charcoal grills. Everyone sat perched in front of their plates waiting for the call to prayer to signal the start of *iftar*, the highly anticipated fast-breaking meal when the sun finally sets.

Ramadan brings a communal change in rhythm. The days are quiet, still, and sleepy until the late morning when neighbors begin emerging from their homes to tend to their gardens, climb into cars, and roll buggies on uneven sidewalks to the markets. The nights are alive with meals eaten with friends in the late evening. Children kick balls and ride bikes with the moon as their flashlight. And a drummer announces the approaching sunrise.

The other week, we were crowded around a circular table where waiters placed in front of us hot plates of chicken kabab and refilled our water glasses. After hearing a little of my husband's and my immigration worries, our friend placed his fork back down on his plate, rested his hands in his lap and said, "Hard times always have a destination."

Usually, when hearing spiritual platitudes by those who are anxious to say something encouraging, my eyes glaze over and my head nods in a polite response. I give the encourager a gentle smile; they're trying to be supportive.

This time though, the words landed a little differently in my ears. Like the falling shapes in a game of Tetris, each word effortlessly locked itself to the next, one on top of the other. As they were released into the air, I felt something in my heart whisper, "Grab onto this. Remember it."

We've spent the last year feeling like we were walking through the valley of the shadow of death. Our days felt like they were decorated more with sorrow than joy. Hope seemed elusive and dwindling. My Bible remained buried in the nightstand, like a too heavy bowling ball, the unturned pages made of lead. I wrestled with the promises written in scripture. Why doesn't God make things right, right now? Here's his chance to do something big and miraculous, but he's quiet.

I've felt huge swells of doubt rise up in me. I've asked questions and received no answer. I've cried out and heard my laments bounce off the walls and return back to me.

Hard times always have a destination.

Those six words spoken across the table over lunch felt like tiny dots pulsing inside me, an ember of hope pushing back the encroaching darkness. They punctuated my skeptical heart, one by one.

I thought about the Turkish drummer, banging loudly in the middle of the dark night. His sole purpose is to alert the town of the coming light, to wake up, to begin preparing the feast. Each knock of the drum shouts out the message, "The sunrise is coming! The sunrise is coming!"

We may be walking through the valley of the shadow of death right now, but God promises to lead us to green pastures and to fields of peace. It may feel like endless midnight but the sunrise is coming.

There is a purpose in the darkness. I may not know what the reason is right now, but I will one day. Consider all the activity that happens when the sun sets and the world becomes dark during Ramadan: meals with neighbors, children playing, feasting, and spending time with family. There is life to be lived in the darkness. There is growth, refinement, and cultivation.

God is certainly not the author of the bad, but he paints beauty out of it. The rays of the rising sun will one day scatter across our valley, sending the dark scurrying away, and things will make sense. All those tattered scraps will be woven into something beautiful.

Not now, but soon.

While we wait for the morning to finally come, we firmly hold on to God's promises and his goodness.

Beautiful things grow in dark places and dawn will always overcome the night.

This comes from Sarah's blog: onefootonboth.com

IN DELIGHT AND YEARNING—I REJOICE

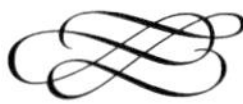

WENDY KONEMANN

My mind gets confused and juggles solitude, loneliness and isolation until they merge into a big blob! Elements of each word merge into the other and, becoming tangled, they land as a blob in my heart.

I married Jeff when I was 20 and he was in the military. We moved often, from one side of the country to the other and 3 years in another country. Brad, our eldest child had gone to 7 different educational institutions and lived in 9 different homes by his first year of high school. He'd been on 33 different flights by the time he was 36 months old as we scurried along after Jeff. I was a desperate connector: "Hello, my name is Wendy and this is my husband Jeff, and these are our three children, Brad, Grant and Laura. We're very nice. We've just moved here. Would you like to be friends? Would you like to come over to dinner? Puff. Puff. Puff." I felt exposed and unsupported in each new place and needed to know I wasn't alone.

When Brad was 12 months old, we had been posted to the other side of the country from my parents and I was stung by a bee. I'd never been stung by a bee before. Jeff was at sea and I phoned my Mum to let her know that I'd been stung by a bee and if I hadn't phoned her that night for her to initiate a rescue operation for Brad…in case I was allergic to bees…in case I'd died. My Mum told me to stop being stupid and that I'd be fine. My heart was hungry for support.

Four years later when living overseas I heard of a military family that had been posted to our host country from the USA. Shortly after arrival, the husband's unit had gone on a military exercise to a country further away for three weeks. The wife, left behind with the 3 small children, suffered a heart attack and died. Their 3 small children starved to death. I cried. My heart broke. I understood.

Jeff eventually left the military and we moved "back home." I hadn't realised how manic I had been in building support around me, until I didn't need to do it anymore. I could walk up the street and wave to my brother as he drove past. Or, say hello to a childhood friend in the store. Extended family everywhere. Isolation had led to loneliness and a need to fill the spaces with people and activity so that I wasn't alone. Solitude was a dirty word.

We have now lived in the same house for 20 years and our children are grown with children of their own. Now I have a yearning for solitude. For time on my own. For space just to be. For a simpler life where every moment isn't filled with doing, achieving, connecting.

So, where has God been during all this time? Present. Always present. I was often so busy making support happen, chasing support, demanding support that I didn't see God in the need. I just needed it to change.

I've chased to have life, to have support, go the way I think it should look. "OK God, this is how it is. This is how I need it to be. Make it happen. Please." Picture fumbling a ball of string or twine that remains just out of reach as your fingers work valiantly to hold it tightly - the more you fumble for it, the more you push it away, forever elusive. All I needed to do was turn into the need and I'd see God there, but I spent so much time chasing for it to be different.

I heard an online sermon on Sunday where the preacher was unpacking The Lord's prayer for us. He asked us what we thought our most audacious prayer was. My mind was filled with audacious requests of my heart's desires.

The preacher then informed us that THE most audacious prayer we could pray was to pray that God's will be done. God's will be done. Phew. That's a pretty scary prayer. For me to pray that prayer with confidence, I'd have to believe, truly believe, that God is good. That God is sovereign. That all the desires that fill my heart are seen and known.

And I'd have to trust that God, who sees and knows, has good plans for my life. That's where the rubber hits the road.

So, in these times of forced isolation due to COVID-19 there's been delight at the forced isolation and solitude, and a yearning for the freedom of movement and connection that I never knew I took for granted until they were taken away from me.

However, in both the delight and the yearning God is present. I have a choice. I always have a choice. I can continue to chase after the things that I want God to be doing, or I can turn to God, in the place of the unmet need and sit at his feet, soaking up his presence, grieving for the yet-to-be-received things that my heart desires, while declaring God's goodness, sovereignty and grace.

Habakkuk 3:17-19

> *Though the fig-tree does not bud*
> *and there are no grapes on the vines,*
> *though the olive crop fails*
> *and the fields produce no food,*
> *though there are no sheep in the sheepfold*
> *and no cattle in the stalls,*
> *yet I will rejoice in the Lord,*
> *I will be joyful in God my Saviour.*
> *The Sovereign Lord is my strength;*
> *he makes my feet like the feet of a deer,*
> *he enables me to tread on the heights.*

When the desires of my heart are not forthcoming, I can either resign myself to it, rebel against it or rejoice through it—putting my trust in God who is all wise, all sovereign.

Today I choose to rejoice.

ABOUT THE AUTHOR

Here is a friend I have yet to meet face to face! I got to know Wendy through her daily postings about her pilgrimage on "El Camino" in Spain. Her deep reflections and insights were a daily inspiration to me during a challenging time in my own life. Her heart for God and the meaning He gives to our lives, through a season of the simple task of walking a pathway toward a spiritual destination—her heart in this—was a light to mine in a time of discouragement. I'm so glad she joined us on these pages of reflection.

INTERLUDE: INVITED

ELLEN JANZEN

When you share your bread
with me
I feel invited to exist.

To live with risk.

When you share your best song
and hold out your arms to dance
I feel invited to delight.

To live with joy.

When you whisper your secret
with a glance into my soul
I am invited to the sacred—
the eternal hope that every living being
is fully formed in beauty.
Invited to magnificence.

To live in wonder—
that each human
holds the imaginative gift of

a life with infinite purpose
that may or may not be
tomorrow's reality.

That the dream of what could be
is surely within each of us
in the secluded alcove we
barely understand
but recognize as our sacred self.

IT WILL BE WORTH IT ALL

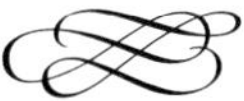

ELLA H.

About 22 years ago, a period of isolation and pain joined forces in my life through a condition I could not grasp and which at that moment had no name. My husband began to experience a huge change in his personality. The change was unpredictable and accompanied by a gradual, increasing pain as well. The ominous name of the change finally surfaced and revealed what was happening—dementia. The journey was slow and long.

Plans could not be made as we did not know what a day might bring. Some days were good. Other days, if someone stopped by or if one of the children visited, he would at times walk away, saying nothing.

Lack of purpose resulted, which was completely out of character. My husband had been a capable, articulate person—interested in everything that involved building. Carpentry, mechanics, anything that could be constructed interested him. He took night school courses every winter.

Now, in the absence of his enthusiasm, depression journeyed with us.

Things that we had made plans for, planned for in our retirement time together, were now put aside. This was a blow to my husband's pride—he had always been a competent, gifted person. He could figure out anything. Now he lived in vulnerability.

Where was I in all of this? Many times feeling isolated and lonely. In that same slot of time, three members of our extended family passed away in the space of three months. One of them was my much-loved sister-in-law. Her loss left a hole in my life.

In addition, I experienced a 20-day hospital stay close to the same time. The prayers of my church family during that illness held onto me. I became very aware that God was still in charge—He does not abandon his children. I learned to look at things in a new way.

The question was no longer "What has been taken?" It became, "What has been left to me?" Yes, God cannot abandon his children. His word is full of precious promises. One that became significant to me was "He preserves my going out and coming in."

I discovered that Jesus is still asking at such times the same question he asked of the blind beggar—"What do you want me to do for you?" (**Matthew 20:34**) He enters into our circumstances in ways we do not comprehend, in ways we don't expect. But he waits for us to invite him in.

How did Jesus enter my circumstances at that time?

As my husband's health declined and he passed away leaving me with many good years ahead, I found that I learned to lean on Jesus and look to him as my daily companion. There was still purpose in the time left for me—I wanted to serve and listen to others who might be suffering in the same way that I had suffered. Sometimes we are inclined to give answers before we have even listened—but I had learned what a gift it was to be heard.

One unexpected and important opportunity came my way two months after my husband's death. An opportunity for which I did not feel qualified in any way, which was starting a Bible study and devotional time at the care home he lived in for his last year. This has continued for the past 8 years. Three friends of like mind go there with me the first Monday of each month. We are blessed each time we go.

There is a chorus that meant a great deal to me during those times when I faced uncertainty and even physical illness. This chorus drew me to look to Jesus. I still sing it once in a while.

"It will be worth it all
when we see Jesus,

each trial will seem so small
when we see Christ.
One glimpse of his dear face
all sorrow will grace
so bravely run the race
til we see Christ."

-by Esther K. Rusthoi (1940)

God's timing and the places He puts us are always good and right. Nearly a decade has passed since these difficulties and I am still discovering how God plans things for our good at this stage of life—But that is another chapter to relate at another time—so stay tuned!

ABOUT THE AUTHOR

Ella has asked to be anonymous as a contributor, so (obviously) I changed her name for this purpose! She is an underestimated octogenarian…with a depth of perspective that makes it a joy to converse with her. She shares from her heart, and always shows heartfelt interest in the person she is with. And one more favourite thing, though maybe there are many still to come… Last time I saw her, she told me she was a little bit naughty when she was a child. She still has that mischievous "little bit of naughty" twinkle in her eye now. I like to think that maybe when I am in my 80s I will be as lively and kind and insightful and "naughty" as Ella.

INTERLUDE: FINDING GOD IN SILENCE

MICHELLE P.

Power cuts. In my part of the world, they are a daily part of life. You know that Zoom call scheduled with your Dad? Yeah, that's tentative because of power cuts. You know that bulk amount of chicken in the freezer? Yeah, you can't depend on it staying frozen because of power cuts. You know that movie you were going to watch on a Sunday afternoon? Or that soup you were going to blend? Or that phone you were going to charge? Or that air conditioner you were counting on for good sleep? Or that science program the kids were going to watch? Or that broken shelf you were going to fix with your drill? Or that cake you were going to bake? Or that fan that was keeping you cool? Or that music you were going to play? Every power cut can feel like a change of plans, or a loss of some kind. Some small, some big.

How do we respond when there are "power cuts"—silence—in our lives? It might be a literal power cut, like in my situation in one of the world's poorest countries. But it might be something else unpredictable that you have gotten used to depending on in your life. It might be a sudden or regular loss. An annoyance. A relationship that comes and goes. A fluctuating bank account. Perhaps this recent COVID-19 lockdown has come with new losses and unpredictability for you, like it has for me.

One of the things that strikes me most in a power cut is the silence—`the quiet that falls on the house when everything else is "unplugged." It strikes me because I didn't realize pre-power cut how much noise was in the background. The fridge, the phone charger, the fan, and some random buzzing from who knows where which has all been silenced. It immediately brings a hush to me for a few minutes (or more!) as everything has suddenly gone quiet.

And then I start hearing things.

I start hearing things that I didn't notice before. The birds. The footsteps. The neighbors. The doors opening. The pouring of water.

So, what's this all about? In silence, we hear things that we didn't hear before. When our world has been "unplugged" we become plugged into something different. We become in tune and more alert to what's around us. Change awakens us. Makes us sensitive. Attentive.

In my years in the desert I have come to see this silence—this period of going unplugged not only from electricity, but also from many other "normal" aspects of life—as an opportunity to listen. To hear. To become attentive to God's Spirit in a fresh way. Every "power cut" in my life is an opportunity to grow in listening and responding to the Father's prompts. What is He saying to me? How is He leading and redirecting my day? What does He want me to let go of and embrace? What does He want me to put away from my thoughts, and take on instead?

When I stop to listen, what is going on in my heart? What am I worried about? What am I thinking about? What is preoccupying my heart? Silence is a great gift for finding ourselves again. For finding God again. For hearing the voices that had grown quiet within us because of the noise outside of us.

I think of silence as a period of fasting. Fasting is something we do out of love for God – periods of time in which we devotedly show Him He is first for us. Times we sacrifice or give up what's "normal" so that we can refocus our hearts and lives on who is most important.

Power cuts might not be a part of your daily life, but what is? What are the irregular things in your "heart-beat" that you're finding challenging to let go of? What does God want to say to you in the "silence" of loss and change?

How could this time of fasting turn to a joyful, deeper walking with Jesus?

"For thus said the Lord GOD, the Holy One of Israel, "In returning and rest you shall be saved; in quietness and in trust shall be your strength." **Isaiah 30:15**

THE FEAST

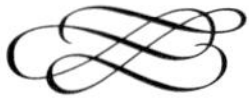

ELLEN JANZEN

It felt like the greatest cost of moving to a new country was the cost to my children.

Week after week, month after month, my heart ached for the things they missed but were slowly forgetting about our life in Canada. Things they missed out on and didn't even know about. People they cried for when I said we lived too far away to go over to visit. Lonely times that would not soon be over.

If I had known more about how resilience develops, I would have worried less. If I had understood the powerful gift of connection, I would have seen the growing delight and joy in each other. The closeness that would become our own version of "us."

But mostly I saw the cost and it scared me. At least this fear served the small purpose of keeping me in God's presence, praying for my children as we muddled our way through the daily challenges of living alone in a city in the North African desert.

As the older two children reached their teen years they found friendships that could be sustained across the distances. Some of those friends lived just a few hours away—we could go for the weekend sometimes and visit. This answered their desire for social connection—and it helped settle my heart, too.

But I still felt sick inside about what they were losing out on—the cost for them of my choice to come here, stay here and let them live "without"—associations, lessons, normal "things" that could make their lives full.

And then one week it all broke apart for me. It's a long story—a series of choices embedded into misunderstandings alongside of crushed expectations and a broken agreement. Long weeks of planning for my daughter to spend time with a good friend who was leaving (permanent loss—again), and a final visit deconstructed for reasons I could not comprehend. Unkept promises and broken hearts.

And I collapsed.

I dissolved in tears that would not stop. Anger, yes. But a steady flow of years of tears that words could not explain. Or fix.

We found other friends to leave our kids with for the day—a consolation for them of sorts, and my husband and I drove to the beach city we often went to for a day "off"—a day of fun and rest. On this day it was an attempt at escape, but there was no fun in it. Just tears and despair. I felt a pounding doubt jarring my soul—uncertainty that I could go on living with this gaping absence of family and church and normal connection and reciprocal care.

My husband and I arrived at our destination as rain began to fall. A sudden cloudburst that fell harder and harder, raindrops bigger than quarters dropping from the sky. We watched the streets washed clean by running streams as we neared the seaside restaurant we loved.

We dashed inside and sat by a window as the river-like streets filled with more water, the level rising with alarming speed. Now, within minutes, the water ran above the edges of car doors—our van just that much higher so our engine stayed dry. "A flash flood," I thought, "this is how this happens."

Thunder cracked overhead in close succession followed by lightning out over the water. Normally I find thunderstorms exhilarating. When a bolt of lightning landed less than a hundred meters from our window, my inner imbalance came together under the arousal of my "flight instincts." There was nowhere to go—no one to turn to. But God.

I turned my heart toward God and whispered—"Okay, you got me. I am listening." And I felt, for a fleeting moment—"This is what Elijah encountered in the storm."

God was in the rain and in the thunder and in the striking light that parted the giant drops of water filling the streets with churning rivers.

But that was not his voice to me.

His voice was barely a whisper and it only said what I already knew. And had forgotten.

"I see you."

It was enough.

I felt my soul fill with the food of the feast laid out—in the presence of all my enemies. My inner warring army of doubting thoughts, resentments, fears and uncertainty. My enemies stopped talking, hushed by the storm.

And my soul feasted. Resting in God's caring gaze.

The next day I read through an entire book I had bought a year earlier but not yet opened. It was the historical narrative of a litany of men and women of God who had marked the world with prayer. Intercessors and mystics whose lives had impacted nations and cities.

Each story carried a single theme: *the cost*. Each one of these Godly characters, these world-moving change agents, had suffered great loss of one kind or another. And in their loss they looked toward God, opened their heart to His presence—invited connection.

And found Him faithful.

"I hear you," I whispered again.

"You see me, and I hear you."

And my soul was restored.

ABOUT THE AUTHOR

Ellen—this is me. I'm Ellen. I think you probably have gotten to know me a little bit through my words. If you want to get to know me more, come for a long visit on my back deck. We can watch the sky until it grows dim. We can sit and talk or be silent. You can tell me what has been challenging in your last year. And I hope that if we meet, you will see something about me that reminds me of you so that we can build on that shared value or strength and become friends.

INTERLUDE: IF IT'S DARKNESS WE ARE HAVING, LET IT BE EXTRAVAGANT

SARAH BAHIRAEI

Sometime after the call to prayer but before any hints of daybreak, I feel her hiccup for the first time. The sliver of moon still glows and so does the green neon sign from the bakery across the street. If the windows were open, the smell of fresh-baked Turkish bread would be floating through.

What a wild thing to feel life moving inside your body.

In the quiet darkness of the not-yet morning and in the warmth of my bed, I rest my hand on the roundness of my abdomen, feeling the pulsing thumps. I reach over to tap my husband awake but his deep, slow breaths remind me it's scarcely 6:30am and I decide to wait.

He had spent all last evening with his head next to my stomach waiting to feel the baby move against his cheek as he murmured a poetic string of Farsi to her into my shirt. "Is it normal?" he looks up, concerned he hadn't yet felt anything. "It's because your voice is calming her to sleep," I reassure him.

It is a certain type of joy to grow any kind of life. It's like spotting a wildflower bursting through the cracks of dried up dirt along the road. When life finds a way to breakthrough, it's a beacon of hope, beauty shimmering in the hard places.

There's a saying from some of the experts in the writing world that says to "write from your scars, not your wounds." The idea behind this being that there is an importance in giving distance to our emotions and experiences before we share. It is vital to respect the process we must go through before broadcasting it to a wider audience.

But what if we don't have the privilege to write from our scars?

We are still very much in the hard stuff of life right now. It's unclear when the new skin will start to form over the hurts and the healing will begin. But perhaps wounds and scarring and hurts and healing don't need to occur independently from each other. Perhaps it is sacred and important when writing transpires from each place side-by-side. Maybe it is good to hold space for both.

This blog is a place where I write from my wounds, despite what the writing experts say. I do it because I don't have the luxury to wait for a scab to grow. The things posted here are raw. It's what we are feeling in real-time. But a tension that comes when drafting each essay is to over-spiritualize the wounds, to end each piece with: This was a hard thing but then we had faith and God changed it! Because God hasn't changed it. Because I haven't gotten the thing for which I have longed. Because there is no guarantee I will get the thing for which I have longed. But there is merit to sharing the waiting and the wrestling and the wounds, even while prayers go unanswered.

Paired with the tension of choosing what to share publicly and what not to share, is the juggling of both the difficulties and the little joys in our life – that little flower growing against all odds amidst the dust and dirt.

It's an inhale of devastating news where the course of our lives takes a neck-breaking turn. It's an exhale of seeing two pink lines appear on a pregnancy test. It's in this space where joy and sorrow share the same breath. It's in buying little white onesies and putting together a crib coupled with long drives late at night with tears as our only prayer because the edges of our world are starting to unravel. The blooming of life and the burying of dreams dance together.

The world's weariness is powerful. It takes strength to push against it and shoulder the door closed. But when it slinks through the bottom gap of the frame and unpacks its bags, hope sits expectantly in the shadows.

Part of what makes hope so elusive is that it must be fought for. It isn't easy or natural to hold on to it in the midst of difficulties because it slips and slides out of our hands as darkness screams louder.

But with the tiny joy of life growing and forming, hope becomes a beacon pointing us ahead, a lighthouse guiding the way forward.

As my belly swells a little rounder with each passing week, and our dresser drawers fill with blankets and pacifiers and diapers, here is what hope is: it's looking onward. It's clinging to that rope — our one and only lifeline — when we can't grip the edge of the cliff any longer. It's resting in that tension and believing there are always miracles tucked away in the darkness.

At the beginning of January, there's always an uptick in blog posts and photo captions about choosing a word for the new year. But how does one determine a word that encapsulates the spirit of the next 365 days? We don't have the luxury to plan for the next rotation around the sun – or even the next month. We live in small seasons, standing at the threshold of the ever-changing day-to-day: face-to-face with life's chaos. It's unclear what tomorrow will be or how things will end.

We wish we had been given a tidier story, one where joy and sorrow don't hold hands, one where dreams bloom and darkness always stays away. I wish we could look down at the healed over scars and think of all the lessons and reflections and gems we gleaned.

But this story is messy and we still have open wounds. Joy and sorrow move in tandem. We can't keep the darkness from entering our lives, but we can hold fast to hope.

We can search for joys glistening through the world's weariness.

And I'll still share here, despite the lack of visible scars, because it's important and beautiful and holy to testify of God's goodness in the midst of waiting for the coming healing.

I didn't choose a word for the new year because I have no idea what the year has in store. But I do know it's bringing hope. It's ushering in joy. It's bringing quiet miracles like the rhythmic hiccups in my stomach in the early hours of the morning.

A baby. A wildflower. Life. It is joy untarnished by the darkness. And, in this new year, may it all be extravagant.

This piece was first published in Sarah's blog: onefootonboth.com

WE FORGET HOW STRANGE WE ARE

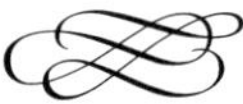

LOUISE C. WOOD, AS TOLD TO ELLEN JANZEN

When I arrived in Central Asia, I chose to live with a family in their traditional home on a lane behind a modern bank. Once I stepped around the well-polished glass windows making up the shiny exterior of the bank, I entered a different world. Here the street was not paved, and the homes did not have modern "luxuries"—things I had always taken for granted—hot running water, electricity, certain kinds of furniture, including beds as I knew them.

Beyond the big gate in a wall facing the street was the central area where fruit trees and grape vines grew—and cars were parked as they arrived. Three rooms had doors off the central open-air courtyard and a separate building that housed a "kitchen" made up the house. It was not the kind of kitchen I was used to, but delicious food came out of that dark little room on a regular basis.

I loved the street food I could get in this city. I'd wait in line for a lovely "samosa" filled with chicken and veggies and then watch while the vendor carefully pulled a page from a book to wrap up my snack. As a book lover, I found the ripping of pages shocking even though they came from books that were no longer valued—books of propaganda dating back a couple of decades to the era of communism. I'd sometimes look down to notice I was holding my snack in the folds of a faded photo of Lenin or Stalin.

I had my own room in this family's home, which already made me "strange" to them, but they quickly became my family there. Part of taking care of me in their culture required them to know where I was at all times. It felt restrictive at first but then I became used to the protection it offered, both realistically and for my reputation in their community. If anything had happened to me, they would have known almost immediately and if anyone in the community had seen me in danger, they would report it to this family. I was "under their wing."

The teenage daughter of the family would come in my room and check out my belongings while I was out—in her culture there was nothing strange or shameful about that. I might even find her wearing something of mine since clothing didn't have a designation to one person the way it does in the west. If I needed my tape or ruler and couldn't find it, she would tell me where it was—which was handy once I got used to the fact that I had to put things I didn't want her to see or use in a locked wardrobe. That was the way to indicate my preference.

The family members slept on bed rolls that were put out each night at bedtime in the two rooms on one side of the central courtyard. By day, one of those rooms was the living room and the other was kept for entertaining special guests—only at night did they become bedrooms.

I was the only one with my "own" room and I did have some choices about that. I chose to have a bed roll like theirs, not so much to be the same but because Western beds were not well made or comfortable. And while it was "my" room, I didn't have the freedom to have my own guests over to visit—that was beyond how their culture worked.

It was normal in this part of the city to have an outhouse in a garden shed instead of a bathroom. The toilet was a hole in the floor—a squat toilet, but the shed doubled as storage and there were building materials and old tyres standing around. There was a tap on the outside wall where I could wash my hands. I got used to this and even became accustomed to using the same old propaganda books as the food vendors in place of toilet paper. Things that would seem wildly strange to my friends at home became somewhat commonplace with time, as I adapted to daily life.

When the family got a copy of the Jesus movie from some other friends, they watched it with great interest and stopped frequently to explain to me exactly what was happening. Many of their explanations started with the phrase, "Did you know…?" I learned lots about the culture and the language by living this way—seeing things through their eyes. It was a unique experience for me as I had never lived outside my own country before this.

We had a lot of laughs when we sat outside in the shady courtyard, which happened often. The mom liked to ask me for words in English—perhaps seeking connection the way I connected to them, through language. She learned the word "chicken" and there was great hilarity when she yelled at her chickens to stay out of her basil and marigolds. She would whip off her scarf and chase them around the yard yelling, *"Chickenlar yemon"*—a mix of English with her own grammatical endings.

When the family had guests or hosted a crowd for a national festival, they needed my room as an extra "guest room" or a prayer room for women. I would move to wherever the "kitchen action" was taking place and participate in preparing food. This was always accompanied by lots of giggles, and it was far more fun to be a part of this than to sit in with all the guests. I started to feel like I really was one of the family.

The experiences of these two years prepared me for other places that I would eventually live. First, I worked in an NGO where the same nationality was found in a neighbouring country—Central Asia is a mosaic of "nations" that sprawl across political borders.

Then I moved to another country that had nothing much in common in terms of language and culture. But the experience of living in a household that watched my every move, considered my property communal and my presence a joy, and included me in their family interaction so closely, prepared me for further cultural "exchange."

The third stop in my international journey was a place where women's lives didn't intersect with the activities outside of the buildings that housed them—with the exception of when they were guests at a wedding. I was the only foreigner living in this mountain city—not only while I was there, but also for as long as anyone could remember. I was definitely far from home when I arrived.

I had been invited into this conservative city on the basis that I would live with a reputable family and teach at a school. My job meant that I could leave the family home each day, but a driver took me between the house and the school. After four months I realized I had never actually put my feet on the ground outside of my own home. The rare times women left their homes their faces were completely covered. I didn't even know my way to the market, or what was on the street out there—a boy came to my door to get my grocery list and then delivered my shopping to me each afternoon.

I did hear about "outside life" from the boys in the English class I was teaching at school. They would come to school each Monday and describe their escapades and bicycle trips over the weekend, and I would listen. I found myself jealous of their freedoms—and resentful on behalf of all these women who would never experience any of these pleasures. Simple joys like feeling the sun on your back, riding along with the wind in your hair.

These women knew how to make the most of every opportunity they got, however. When a wall between homes was demolished and re-built, there was a series of tea parties with neighbours who had no other spontaneous way of being in contact with each other once that wall went back up. The joy they found in two weeks of connection made up for the months when having tea together required considerable planning. I marvelled at their resilience.

Periodically I would take the train out of town and down from the mountains to visit the capital city. Leaving the train station when I arrived there was always a jolt into reality. I found myself surprised and almost overcome with the weight of making each decision for myself. Suddenly I had to commandeer a taxi and get myself safely to a hotel, completing the evening by obtaining a meal for myself from a local restaurant. The list of decisions felt overwhelming after living in such a sheltered, restrictive way.

My expectations of myself and others had gradually changed over the months of living "in seclusion." Sometimes I was surprised by my own reaction because I didn't realize that I had gotten used to a new way of doing things.

Eventually, when my time in the mountains came to a close, I moved down to that city and for the first six months, I felt like I was on a perpetual holiday. I could go out whenever I chose and there were even gardens I could wander through, as slowly as I wished. I felt like a bird that had found the door to her cage left open. So long as I was home by nine in the evening, I was a "free bird."

By contrast, there were other foreigners who found their life in the big city annoyingly restrictive. They sometimes complained about the very things I found so freeing—to them being out on the street no later than nine in the evening was a hardship.

So, coming "home" to England in between work assignments in these far-off cities started, not surprisingly, to feel less and less familiar to me. I would come to visit my family and find that I had less in common with them and my friends than was comfortable. I sometimes wondered how to fit in, and I missed that feeling of belonging that comes when you live and work abroad.

The restrictions that came with the pandemic were as much a surprise to me as they were to anyone. I had been in England for several months and had found a place to live in a large communal house with nine other people. We realized that COVID-19 was a threat but with so little warning, we didn't see it changing our daily lives.

I watched as my housemates adjusted to the restrictions, thinking to myself—"This is taking me back to what I am used to." Expectations dictate how we respond to most things, and from my history of living in places where I had less personal freedom, this was not a hardship. I could still do more things than I had done in some of the places I had lived. One night I told my housemates the story of the outhouse and our propaganda books for toilet paper. They looked at me with a little confusion and one of them said, "Sorry—was that something YOU did or a story you heard?" I saw in their surprised faces the long journey that had taken me far into another culture—I felt pretty strange in that moment, despite that the whole world had been thrown out of what makes sense to us.

But I knew how to give myself a sense of purpose which was so helpful for my sanity. I found an NGO where I could help be a part of the provision for those who were truly suffering from lack of food, and each morning I was able to work as a volunteer.

I feel like I am investing in my roots here in the city I grew up in once again, in a time when the crisis has been a great equalizer. It has offered me the opportunity to be useful in circumstances to which I have the skills to adapt. Living overseas teaches you to hold almost everything—time, language, cultural norms—in the context of adaptation. There is always some deeper nuance or meaning that you catch on to as you live there for a while.

It has been harder to watch my parents, who have been fiercely independent until now, having to adapt. They are not free to leave their house, and I do their grocery shopping and delivery for them. They struggle to accept this new role of depending on me, but they need to in order to keep their health protected. It isn't the same as cultural protection the way I've experienced it, but the limits are remarkably similar.

One day, recently, I stood in line for an hour waiting for prescriptions for my parents to be filled. People around me commented and complained about the long wait—they were used to being able to come in and pick up prepared medications within minutes. Standing in line was an unusual hardship for them. I realized again, how I had become used to any kind of bureaucratic activity taking hours if not days. One hour of waiting in a queue seemed minimal and still within my expectations of efficiency. Someone commented on my "patience" and I reflected that I am not really patient at all. I just have different expectations in these circumstances.

And maybe most importantly, everything I learned about praying in times of adjustment has come back to carry me forward with hope. I have no idea how long this time of "lockdown" will continue. But I've become more used to the reality that I have no idea what will happen next. I have to live in the moment I've got and trust that God has the bigger plan in his hands—and I depend on Him for the next door to open. Whenever that might be.

ABOUT THE AUTHOR

Louise is a long-time friend… I am not sure when and where I first met her. She lives with one foot always close to the edge of uncertainty. I'm not sure if she will stay in one city or country long enough for me to get there to see her…and I admire her for it. She has taught me to pay attention to the signs all around us that God and his angel servants are nearby. Her awareness of this is the strength she lives by. We see each other somewhat regularly, one way or another, and each time we get to share our lives over a cup of coffee, tea or Asian soup, I leave the encounter with a feeling of delight. It is a gift to call Louise my friend.

INTERLUDE: SHINING FACES
MICHELLE P.

How can we find God in isolation?

Isolation will mean different things for different ones of us.

For some of us it is being crammed in a small space with our children and with our work and trying to navigate chaos.

For others of us, it's the silence, the stillness, the loneliness that has suddenly come upon our lives. For some of us it might involve ailment, sickness and feeling alone in our pain.

I like to think of isolation as an invitation. An invitation from God; a period of fasting. A period when we don't have what is normal, we don't have our normal supports, our normal schedules, our normal jobs and we enter a time of growing closer to him.

When the river has been dammed, the water dries up. What do we do in the middle of a dry riverbed where there is still water for us?

There's an invitation from God to sink our roots deeper to tap into that unlimited water source.

God uses isolation again and again in the Bible to prepare his people for what's to come.

Joseph was in isolation in prison, far away from anyone who shared his faith and he had no idea how long his isolation would last. He had no input from anyone other than God's Spirit and the words passed down from generations by his father and grandfather.

It was his faith in God that sustained Joseph through that time of isolation and prepared him for a purpose—to save Egypt and Israel and many other nations. And from that time, he was exalted from out of the pit and prison. God moved him to a place of influence and honour and usefulness for God's glory. God uses isolation to prepare his people for His purposes.

Moses experienced isolation on the mountain and came out with a shining face.

There is hope for us in isolation.

To find God, to find Jesus.

John the Baptist was in isolation and came out ready for his ministry. Jesus experienced temptation 40 days in the wilderness. The experiences of isolation were a doorway to his ministry which changed the world for history.

And there are many more stories of great leaders in the Bible—most of them experiencing some form of isolation and finding God's presence there at a time in their formation.

What could God do in us if we respond to this isolation as a gift, as an invitation to know him more; to embrace the silencing and the changes of our lives, to let him transform and redeem the uglier parts of us that we don't like that come out in these stressful times.

What could God do in us if we surrender to him in this time and embrace it?

This time could change our church, our life, and our nation.

What an opportunity to respond to God, to know our best friend, Jesus, in these hard times and to walk closely with him.

Maybe our faces will be shining when we come out of it.

I sure hope so.

THE BROKEN POT

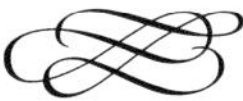

AIMEE ROOF

Smack, his knee suddenly hit the back of my head. The blow came from behind, unexpected. I fell forward, surprised… Standing near a swing-set, he had underestimated his strength and didn't see me. A hit I did not see coming—sounds a bit like life.

In saying yes to going abroad, I experienced that there are some losses and changes I could have prepared for, but there are unexpected hits, losses that one can't prepare for.

Loss of normal, loss of nearness to family, loss of friends as distance and time apart grows. Isolation, when I would have experienced connectedness. However, after years of adjusting and becoming a part of a community, my hardest journey was in leaving the field.

With any transition come uncountable secondary losses — loss of a sense of purpose, a sense of home, familiarity and participating in my new culture and language, celebrations of new holidays, and new traditions. I knew I was signing up for hardship and possibly death, but death to self looks and feels much less glorious. Some of my losses were: loss of a man I loved, a dream of our ministry together, my current ministry relationships, my team that had become family, passport and visa issues. This came with trauma, isolation and the feeling of shame.

A month before these big losses began and other hurts followed, I was sitting in a garden, connecting with the Lord, contemplatively enjoying the scenery. All of a sudden, a gardener appeared. He was tending to some potted plants a short distance away.

I saw him pull out a chisel, a tool for breaking the terra cotta pot that held a little pine tree. The little tree was rootbound and the gardener broke open the pot... Crack, it was sudden. A perfectly good pot was smashed. Why would you break such a thing? This felt significant to me as I watched, like something a prophet of the Bible would have seen, happening in front of my eyes.

Then the gardener placed the tree into the dirt of a bigger pot.

Some of the weak foundations around my identity had interpreted events as possibly something God caused or allowed to happen. Was He the gardener in this parable? I wanted to be near Him but didn't know if I could trust Him or others.

My first step out of this feeling of isolation was intimacy with the Lord. I tentatively pressed in and heard "I am here, I took all the pain on the cross, give it to me. I can take it. Press into my love, press into my face, press into what I offer. I am here for you." This feeling of intimacy was steadying, the years of foundation we had built could sustain me through life's hits. He was guiding me out of a victim mind-set. Grace gave me the gentle way of humility to move forward. Not "to-do's" or spiritual hoops, but a pressing into the greater tangible life and connectedness He offered.

Times of solitude and silence became consistent life-sources, allowing me to encounter Jesus and see my actual state, the me going through these things. In my departure from my country of service, I traveled to another country to debrief. In this time, I saw afresh the kindness of Jesus. It was the same me, in the same place I had served short-term 10 years prior, some of the same local friends who had vibrant lives in the Lord. And this loud cheer, as it were, from the host of heaven. I had traveled so far from home for so many years and yet was still so near to the Lord.

This was a taste of the heaven, the cloud of witnesses cheering the Lord's people on as I was unraveling the trauma and loss I had experienced. In debriefing my last year, a man in a small group listened to my story and as he looked at me with kindness, I saw anew the face of our compassionate Jesus.

I would like to share another big step. In my first year back in the US, an unlikely spot in my plans, a ministry school in Northern California, I had many encounters with the Living Good Father, He changed everything. He renamed me, as the scripture says this land is now called Married.

"You will be a crown of splendor in the LORD's hand, a royal diadem in the hand of your God. No longer will they call you Deserted, or name your land Desolate. But you will be called Hephzibah, and your land Beulah; for the LORD will take delight in you, and your land will be married." - **Isaiah 62:3-4**

He reframed His goodness to His character, not the events in my life.

After refilling myself with so much truth, one day I woke up happy, a slightly estranged emotion. Hope continued to grow. Again, not hope in circumstances, but that God's goodness would look after me all my days.

In preparation for my second year of continuing in ministry school, the Lord gave me a dream. In it a pastor I knew, told me "the biggest obstacle for next year was not finances" (something I had concern over, not knowing how another year in the USA would be possible). As I awoke, I felt the dream was God speaking. I asked God what the two obstacles were—"anxiety and loneliness" were the two words resounding in my heart.

Another big step forward. Anxiety and loneliness, emotions yes, yet they presented choices of how I could view things. No matter the season or circumstances, the world faces loneliness, mine I masked by other things. These were things to do, successes, or little joys—each thing seemed to hide a gaping hole that was inside of my heart. They took me away from feeling my pains or realities.

Face to face contemplative prayer and encountering the Lord's face helped me see Christ more clearly, and then myself. I recognized that subtle, cultural messages were a powerful force—but not all Kingdom values. Scripture recalibrated my values to the Lord's thoughts, not the pervading cultural messages.

I slowly let trusted friends into my hurts, my process, receiving freedom as I shared, displacing shame. I declared scriptures and truths, like "Through Jesus, I am 100% loved and worthy to receive all of God's blessings" (see *Colossians 1:12-14*). Declarations and thanksgiving changed my perspectives.

David used five stones to take down Goliath. The five stones for victory the Lord gave me this year were intimacy, faith, confidence, wisdom, and peace. I come out of this season with great confidence that could only be built on a stronger foundation: a way of seeing that God is bigger than the circumstances, simply His character pointing to goodness.

Resilience—with joy—has grown in the face of trials. Essentially, I know that no matter what happens I will be ok and intimately connected with the Lord. When I experience "hits," I know a way forward, into His heart and truth. My pain had a purpose and God's goodness brought me into the fulfillment of the promises of Psalm 23—a resting place, soul refreshing, and a feasting in the face of enemies.

We can declare with confidence, "Surely your goodness and love will follow me all the days of my life, and I will dwell in the house of the Lord forever."

ABOUT THE AUTHOR

Aimee was walking through a long valley of painful loss when a mutual friend introduced us. As we talked a sense of understanding emerged…and then deepened through both words and silence over time spent together. She faced her heartache head on and with determination put one foot in front of the other, sounding unsteady and yet fully trusting God—both at the same time. She moved forward to the sunlit meadows at the end of her valley and began to blossom—as if she was a tree that had come out of a deep winter with her roots burrowed into the unseen source of life. I was lucky to be her friend during this season. With every fibre of her self, and with every word she speaks, her "being Aimee" reminds me that God is faithful.

INTERLUDE: EVERLASTING ARMS UNDERNEATH YOU

ELLEN JANZEN

All those stories.

How many billions of people lived on this earth before we even arrived? And each one had a story—with interest and adventure, challenge and triumph, defeat and sorrow—woven into a pattern completely their own. A story that carried them from birth to death.

And yet, still, my story is unique. Uniquely unique.

And, no matter how you are feeling today—your story is just as incredible and purposeful and precious as mine or anyone else's.

When we stop to think of the "greats" of our time, I always go pretty directly to Mother Theresa. Who somehow managed to end her life quietly, in the shadow of the uproar caused by Princess Diana's death. Just as she lived, she left inconspicuously after a lifetime of great deeds.

Mother Theresa was surely one of the most admirable, God-focused women of all time.

But the point of her story wasn't about herself. The point was and still remains simply this: every single story, no matter how shabby the body that carries it—every single one matters. Every single fading, dying body is worthy of dignity and yes, each one matters.

Whoever you are, whereever you are, whatever has gone on in these months in your life—however shabby your life feels in these moments of uncertainty or stress or loss or collapse—this is for you.

As much as any life matters, as much as any of us has purpose, whatever the prize is—you are worthy. You matter.

What matters to you is of infinite interest to the God of the heavens who is your maker. Don't let anyone—especially your own self—tell you that you don't count. Because you do.

God sees you and counts you as precious. And here is what He has for you today:

> *There is no one like the God of Jeshurun,*
> *who rides across the heavens to help you*
> *and on the clouds in his majesty.*
> *The eternal God is your refuge,*
> *and underneath are the everlasting arms.*
> *He will drive out your enemies before you,*
> *saying, 'Destroy them!'* **Deuteronomy 33: 26, 27**

To whatever extent you are able, let your whole self—heart, mind, soul, spirit and body—let your whole self rest on his everlasting wings. He fights for you. He is near.

LOVING MORE THAN DOING

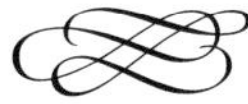

NADIA M.

In my first month of living in my new village, one big goal was achieved. I found a friend close to my age who agreed to be my language helper. It marked the first chapter of my life here with a small triumph.

This small town, my new home, was made of low buildings and tall caves. There was no sea here, just rocks and hills and a group of numerous people for me to get to know. Adapting to this change takes effort—surrendering to God through prayer and patience. And having strength to ask for help again and again. Knowing nothing, it seems, and hoping it will get better.

I had already lived in this part of West Asia for over a year, in a big city, modern and comfy—lots of shops, easier transportation, and the Sea. So close to the sea, one of my favourite things. Life there lacked a social element of a community to be a part of. So the move was needed—I couldn't survive with just the sea, by myself.

Finding Gamze, who would teach me Turkish, was my first gift. She lived in a beautiful home with her parents, in a middle class neighbourhood within walking distance. They looked like a harmonious and content family to me and I was happy to begin my "language learning journey" in their home, becoming in some way a part of a local family—an important step toward being known in the community here.

After each two-hour language lesson, Gamze was predictable—"Would you like to drink tea with us?" We would move to her mom's domain, the kitchen where I would sit on the couch by their dining table and sample home-made goodies and drink a cup of Nescafe that I really didn't care for. Especially not in August. Or we would drink cup after cup of tea that Gamze served me for a couple of hours, my tired brain struggling to take in more language, while secretly wishing to go home and rest.

Not accepting the invitation to stay for tea, especially at the beginning, would be rude in this culture—it would mark me as an outsider. And by staying, I became a member of their family. Gamze and her mom, a housewife, would kiss my cheeks and hug me tight each time I came or left again. They felt free to touch my hair or caress my cheek, telling me how sweet I was to them—something I really missed as an Italian girl from a town where physical contact is normal.

One day the hot weather of August sucked all the motivation out of me and I went down to their house feeling pretty empty inside. I didn't want to deal with language that day. I remember thinking to myself, "Why am I even going there today? I have nothing to offer—I can't talk about Jesus and I don't have any positivity left. My words are limited…" Everything felt so difficult. Yet I prayed for strength especially for the time for tea, after the lesson.

During our lesson Gamze and I slipped into a chatting time for about 15 minutes— a time when we forgot about grammar and structure and mixed our shared languages together…and thoughts from our hearts. Though we had never spoken about private or deep things before, on this day we shared deeply about relationships.

I felt a nudge inside of me—"Nadia, if you desire her to open her heart to you in a deeper friendship, you have to share first. You open up too and lead the way." So I spoke of the last relationship I had left, the painful ending. After that, Gamze shared with me that she was in a relationship that I viewed as seriously complicated. As she shared, God gave me the wisdom to respond simply but with understanding. This chat was changing how my day was going and opened the door for our friendship to step into a new place. From this day on our friendship went deeper.

The kitchen is not far from the room where we have our lesson and we can usually hear Gamze's mom cleaning, cooking or talking to another daughter who lives in another town. As we came out of the lesson room on that day I was greeted as usual with "How are you sweetie? Come and sit down!" Which, of course, I did. But on this day we didn't have the soup or the sweets that they so often have ready. We just drank tea.

I was still new in the house and I had not really met Gamze's dad. I would greet him in passing and had observed that he seemed like a good dad, providing for his family. So as we sat there that day I decided to ask more about the family and I thought to say, "How did your mom and dad meet?" I surely couldn't have imagined the reality I was about to hear.

Gamze started with, "My dad and mom are the fruit of marriages that came from a population exchange that happened in 1924."[1] Their parents, as a result, set up an arranged marriage for them. Gamze told the story to me like this:

"When my mum was 16 years old, her family was struggling financially so her mom gave her in marriage to the son of a far off relative. My mum didn't like him and she didn't want to get married so young, but she had no choice. Her sisters were married off in the same way. Their brother, the only son, was worthy of good care, a college education and he was the only child allowed to marry whomever he chose.

"My parents never had a happy marriage—my dad was selfish and rude, never caring to spend time with his daughters, me and my sisters. He didn't talk kindly with us or encourage us, especially when we started to study at university. We dreamed of becoming someone one day. Lately he has been so angry and we don't know what to expect. When he explodes my mom just cries.

"I don't love him, I can't wait to find a good job and have the independence to leave this house." With these last words, tears streamed down her face. It was the first time she allowed me to see her vulnerability. She must have felt my empathy for her and felt safe to share this.

I was deeply touched by her trust and my heart filled with compassion. I come from a broken family and longed many times to have an engaged and kind dad. In that moment I felt a covering of wisdom and divine strength come over me. I followed the conversation using a combination of English and the local dialect.

I hardly said a word as Gamze poured out her heartache for me to hear and see what she had suffered. My role was to give her a place to open her heart. I felt in those moments that I had been sent by God, as the instrument of His presence, to hear her sorrow on this specific day. She didn't need my opinions or an effort to fix her, and she especially didn't need me to say what the neighbours around her would have said, "Don't cry, you'll feel better. You'll get out of here and things will turn out fine."

There was such satisfaction in being able to do this—to sit and listen and care. Only at the very end of her talking, I shared a few words, some of my family history and the pain I could relate to so well. She seemed surprised that what I had appeared to be was not necessarily so—a young single woman working in a foreign country most people would assume I came from a perfect, or near perfect family.

I heard myself say, "I learned from my own life experience that our parents are not perfect and yes, they have done wrong things—things that caused us pain. But in God I found a perfect Father, and in fact he has been like a dad and a mom to me. I hope you can experience this one day and know him as I have. I will pray for your dad. God listens to our prayers when we cry out to him."

At about this time, Gamze's mom came into the kitchen and found us deep in conversation which Gamze quickly summarized for her. She included the part about my family and how I understood the heartache they carried. Gamze's mom busied herself making tea, looking intensely toward me from time to time.

When she finally spoke, she echoed Gamze's response, "You know it was not easy for me to marry this man my mom chose for me. I just had to accept him as my husband. Life with him has not been easy, especially when we had three young daughters and were living in a big old house, managing a wine factory. I worked hard and did my best to be present, a good mom to my daughters. I told myself that what happened to me would not happen to them. It was not possible for me to get a driver's license or study for a degree or to have a personal income that could give me independence.

But I fought for my daughters and prayed that they would go to university and be a somebody, whether they married or not. I wanted my daughters to be able to get a job and be independent."

As she said this, Gamze's mom started cry. I had seen her be emotional before—she was a generous and kind woman, regularly calling her mom and sisters and daughters, making sure each one was doing okay.

Even though she has gone through so much in life she laughs loudly at the fun things in life and cries with people when things are hard. I love her good heart and her sensitivity to others. I love the way she treats me as if I was her daughter.

With Gamze's help, the mom went on, "This last period has been especially hard. I thought my husband was improving and getting softer and quieter as he got older, but he has changed back again. He complains about the grocery shopping and about what I cook and about the things that Gamze and I need."

Once again, I didn't know what to say but felt I just needed to listen and be the ears that heard their story. All I could offer was, "I will pray for him and for you. Thank you both for sharing so much with me." With appreciation in her voice, she turned to Gamze and said, "She is like an angel sent to our house."

At the door they hugged me goodbye. I reminded them, "I will pray for him." As they waved goodbye and watched me leave I noticed their faces bore wide smiles and looked much brighter.

I walked home in a cloud of joy, my heart swelling with what I had learned. These hours had been a lesson much bigger than language or culture. I had learned that God can use me on the days when I feel I have nothing to give. Even when I am struggling to function in my 2nd and 3rd languages, He has a purpose. I don't need to "have it all together" in order to sit down and listen and be a friend.

The verse that came to mind to encourage me was the one from *2 Corinthians 4:7-10*:

> *"But we have this treasure in jars of clay to show that this all-surpassing power is from God and not from us. We are hard pressed on every side, but not crushed; perplexed, but not in despair; persecuted, but not abandoned; struck down, but not destroyed. We always carry around in our body the death of Jesus, so that the life of Jesus may also be revealed in our body."*

I identified fully with this image—I was just a clay jar. It reminded me deeply that the power belongs to God and is not reliant on my ability. God had brought me to that house as His instrument of love in order to give significance to these women through telling their story. He can use me or not, on any given day. But I also learned that deep understanding and friendship doesn't get rooted if we just talk about beautiful things or if we "wear the facade" of foreigners who have it all together.

Deeper friendship with Gamze and her mum continued to grow and a few days later the mum told me, "Nadia, your prayers worked. My husband has become more settled and quiet. Thank you so much." And she continued to ask for my prayers for other things as well, saying "God hears and accepts your prayers."

Once I had finished doing language study with Gamze, I continued to visit with the family—spending long hours in the kitchen, sometimes over cups of tea or delicious food they had prepared. We talked sometimes about spiritual matters, but in the end, they were not pursuing further understanding of God for themselves. I don't know what the spiritual value will be of what we shared—sometimes we just drink tea and watch TV, but I believe I have planted seeds by listening to their stories.

A believing friend who has lived here for many years explained that often we don't get to see those seeds being nurtured. "Even though you don't see the fruit of your ministry, God calls you to be faithful. The result always depends on Him and comes from His timing."

I recalled these words when I was struggling to find my sense of purpose. Through this conversation I began to realize that God wants my love first and the rest will come as a result of the loving relationship I have with Him. Many people think our first job is to talk with people about God, making those conversations happen every day, somehow working toward that and that alone. But loving God is the first thing Jesus asked of us—and it was so important for me to come to recognize this is my "calling"—my work. Loving God is my service.

Between August 2019 and March 2020 when the lockdown for COVID-19 took place, I got busy in my life with all manner of things, adapting to a new pace of living and meeting people. My times with God were one of the "things" I had on a to-do list for each day. I didn't realize at the time, but mainly I was keeping up with a task, not enjoying a relationship with him.

Each day I set time to pray, worship, listen to songs and read—all of which helped me face the day better. It kept me from feeling God might be mad (or get mad) at me. Looking back, I can see I was not feeling renewed, fulfilled or delighted by spending that time with God—experiencing His presence.

I was in a place of condemnation because my lack of connection in my devotional time was leaving me with a lot of silence. I would think "I can't hear God's voice because I don't know how to stay well with him in my personal time, but God why don't you speak louder? You could allow me to hear you easily. I need you to tell me something clear in this and that. Why do you let me go into my day with no answers, or into a struggle or situation with no answers? Is the problem me or you?"

The main obstacle was my focus—His silence. At the same time, I was easily distracted by many other thoughts. If I was intentional and disciplined, I could stick to a routine of reading, prayer and listening to songs, but most days I was in a rush to get on with my day.

I had lost a previous habit of singing and dancing in my time with God because my neighbour had told me she could hear my singing and her husband commented that my songs were Christian. I thought it didn't matter if I gave this up—it was more important that my neighbours not be disturbed or annoyed by my expression of a faith that was different to theirs.

There were, of course, sweet moments when I felt encouraged by a song or a verse. Some of these moments happened alone and others when I was worshipping with my team—but they were fleeting. I was not living from an emotional connection to God.

Restrictions for COVID-19 arrived here just as close friends left for a time away. Others left because of travel warnings. It was an intense week with things changing quickly and a sense of powerlessness taking over even daily routines.

The changes forced me to look more intentionally at my personal time with God. I was no longer able to ignore what was going on or pretend to myself that it would all be okay and would get better on its own. I had been telling myself that structure was good, that I didn't need the personal nature of singing and dancing, and that He would be here with me, loving me through these activities.

I realized that I wanted freedom and intimacy with God—that my heart matters to Him. I needed to actually experience His presence in my own soul.

Miraculously, at exactly the right time, I found a Member Care person I could easily talk to. Her insights and ideas for connecting with God brought it all together. Something clicked inside me, and the amount of time available due to lockdown helped me spend more time in creative expressions of worship. God redeemed the limitations and the COVID-19 crisis turn out for good for me.

My focus has shifted away from the problem of "not hearing His voice." I'm able to accept silence knowing that even if I hear nothing in my personal time with God, He writes something of substance, something tangible, into my spirit, while I may not even be aware of it. There is a song that says, "Even when I don't see it, you are working. Even when I don't feel it, you are working, you never stop working."

With this I also feel much less rushed. A thousand thoughts don't crowd into my head at once. I can sit and be still and spend time with God however I want to. Sometimes I just sit, but I also feel free to sing—so I do. If I want to write things down, I do. Sometimes I draw. If I feel a dance, then I dance.

The condemnation I was feeling is gone—what I felt from God and from myself. I am grateful for how alive I feel in my spirit. I think the decision to sing and dance despite being heard by my neighbours "shouted" down the enemy and quickly brought me to freedom.

I am finding myself again. I am discovering new things about my identity and intimacy I was made to have with my Father. I am exploring the natural connection and discovering healing in His presence and restoration. It is all bringing me healing. I can't explain how this journey brought me so radically into a new space—apart from His divine work.

I feel His presence in my life. Knowing that He is doing this in my life, I trust Him —I'm held in His hands. How beautiful you are Lord!

---

1. https://en.wikipedia.org/wiki/Population_exchange_between_Greece_and_Turkey

ABOUT THE AUTHOR

How am I so lucky and blessed to have met so many strong women and seen their hearts, so raw while at the same time so beautiful with courage? Nadia is this kind of gem. Soon after I met her, she let me put my arms around her, as if she was my precious daughter or niece, and she wept. It was a sacred moment of letting God's work come through a flood of healing tears. It takes great courage to be so honest with our own pain—but then, out of these moments, we carry healing to others. Nadia carries these gifts with a gentle smile and her beauty is a shining light that brings me joy. I am so blessed.

INTERLUDE: FEELING USELESS

ELLEN JANZEN

One of my favourite writers on the spiritual journey is Henri Nouwen. He has a way of articulating lessons my heart is learning, usually at a snail's pace. His words make me feel I am pursuing something valuable—that my slow progress is worthwhile.

It is good to be "not alone" in this journey. Through the words he has authored, Henri Nouwen has become a friend, a companion in my search for meaningfulness—which gives me courage.

Today we, Henri and I, had a conversation of sorts over the topic of feeling useless…which has been a battle for me many times in my life.

During this time of quarantine and restriction, I've noticed the futility we feel when we can't "get things done" the way we would like to. Some of my family members have lost their jobs or clients. It is hard to give up the busyness and meaningful activities of life that we are used to—or that provide a way to pay the bills.

Sometimes the "uselessness" or helplessness against the circumstances of life puts us into a different posture before God. Paradoxically, being "useless" might actually turn out to be quite a useful space—the exact place to prompt growth.

Often I find myself in a wrestling match before I am able to put my cares and feelings into the hands of God. It often takes a cliff wall to get me to take a look inside my soul. I avoid disturbing my sense of equilibrium—until I have to.

It takes a bit of reflection to push through to the place where I can trust that the current dis-ease and the concern for the future are not mine to control. I have choices to make, but they aren't in control of what happens next. Often the biggest choice is to keep on trusting that God is for me…and that He is good.

When I push into that place, there is a tranquility and peace that restores me. Restores my soul, "beside quiet waters," as Psalm 23 says.

Maybe God welcomes those times when we are "down" in a valley of struggle— where we feel useless or unproductive. Maybe getting lost is really a part of finding His pathway for our hearts to follow. Maybe the feeling of being useless is supposed to help us find out more about ourselves, and in the process more about God.

Henri Nouwen helps me think more deeply and pursue God's presence more fully…

"It indeed is a hard discipline to be useless in God's presence and to let him speak in the silence of my heart. But whenever I become a little useless I know that God is calling me to a new life beyond the boundaries of my usefulness."[1]

Henri seems to anticipate that there is something bigger about to happen. Something good. Those are big drops of courage to my soul—falling in through the cracks in my invisible ceiling.

I find myself shift, reflecting bravely…hoping for good growth, stronger roots.

Thanks, Henri, for the good talk today. You've carved paths for us in the unknowns when we find our lives turned upside down—and we are grateful.

In case you would like another round of conversation with Henri Nouwen, I will include this longer quote from this book.

> Prayer is not a way of being busy with God instead of with people. In fact, it unmasks the illusion of busyness, usefulness, and indispensability. It is a way of being empty and useless in the presence of God and so of proclaiming our basic belief that all is grace and nothing is simply the result of hard work. Indeed, wasting time for God is an act of ministry, because it reminds us and our people that God is free to touch anyone regardless of our well-meant efforts. Prayer as an articulate way of being useless in the face of God brings a smile to all we do and creates humor in the midst of our occupations and preoccupations.

Thinking about my own prayer, I realize how easily I make it into a little seminar with God, during which I want to be useful by reading beautiful prayers, thinking profound thoughts, and saying impressive words. I am obviously still worried about the grade! It indeed is a hard discipline to be useless in God's presence and to let him speak in the silence of my heart. "But whenever I become a little useless I know that God is calling me to a new life beyond the boundaries of my usefulness.[2]

---

1. Henri Nouwen, *You are the Beloved: Daily Meditations for Spiritual Living*, New York, Convergent, 2017, p 147.
2. Nouwen, *You are the Beloved*, p. 147.

BRING IT ON

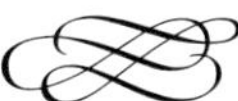

SHARON MACDONALD

For over ten years, I have lived a steady schedule where I blend a life of adventure as a flight attendant—flying around the continent and occasionally further—with a quiet life at home between flight "pairings." I love both the newness of visiting cities I've never been to, and the steady predictability of life at home.

My daily life before COVID-19 was an even mixture of the two aspects, alternating travel with being at home every other week. On the weeks I was home, I would play "catch up." Catch up on laundry, on visiting my children and grandchildren, and spending the weekends with my husband when he was home from being on the road all week. I would catch up with friends and family abroad.

There would be quilting and housework, gardening (indoors or out) and cooking. There was the occasional visit to the hair dresser, or the doctor's office, or a dental checkup and Church attendance on Sunday mornings and small group meetings on Thursday nights when I wasn't flying somewhere for work.

All these things gave a sense of regularity in my days. Although each day was different from the day before, the weeks and months worked their way into a predictable pattern. God was a part of my day, but because I could be working any time around the clock, my devotions weren't any particular time of the day. I would read something from the Bible in the morning, and more often than not, have a longer time reading or listening to my Bible app in the evening when I would go to bed. I always prayed in the shower, so no matter what time I slept or woke in the day, always shower time given to God.

Over the years my fluid schedule became a comfortable and fulfilling mix of these two sides of my life.

My husband, who hauled fuel and was also away from home a fair bit of the time, often commented on how both of our jobs, his with a big company and mine with a top Canadian airline, were quite recession-proof. He has been a dangerous goods trucker for 13 years, and I have been with my company for more than 13 years. We felt our jobs were secure. He said, "People won't stop driving, and they won't stop flying."

Well, those jobs may have been recession-proof, but apparently they weren't COVID-19-proof.

He was the first to be out of work. It felt strange in the month of March to get in my uniform and pack my bags for the week, while my husband stayed home. It was our first role reversal. Usually I'd say goodbye to him on Monday evenings, when he would go to the truck yard and be away for the next 5 days.

If I was working that week, I would always try to "bid" for my schedule to go away and come back while he was away. He would never know I was gone.

But now things were different. I worked every week that I could. I didn't know how much longer we would be flying with the pandemic warnings suggesting travel was one of the main culprits in spreading the virus. It wasn't long before I found out. During the third week in March I got a letter asking if I wanted to pick one of four options, which included the option to retire, or go on a one-, two-, or three-month leave of absence.

I only had a few hours to make my decision as I would be flying when the deadline came. It was a decision I never thought I would have to make. I was not prepared for this. I thought I had been at the company long enough to evade any possibilities of leaving permanently, or even temporarily.

I had worked briefly for Thomas Cooke. I loved that airline. I loved its people! I was shocked when they closed their doors. It was the first time I thought that this could happen to anyone. Given Canada's small airline market, I didn't think it would ever happen here.

Spiritually, I felt like my life was going along splendidly. I am happily married. We have a small nest egg. Our children are grown and doing very well (although, only the Lord knows what's in their hearts). We have grandchildren that we live close to, and love to death!

We knew what it was to live poor in the early years of our marriage, and Calgary has certainly treated us better than that. We haven't been to the food bank since we moved out here 15 years ago. As a matter of fact, I don't know how many times I have grocery shopped for people and just dropped off boxes of food at someone's house, or left bags of donations on my doorstep for pick up. I used to be the one looking for the donations to come to clothe my children.

For all intents and purposes, life has been good to us here.

Then came COVID.

It reminds me of a time a year ago. I was walking along a cement path from one building to another. A group of us were walking together. I had walked this path many times. I knew it was just a short section that was cement and the rest was either gravel covered pavement or rough, broken up parking lot. It was on the cement that I caught my toe just on the lip of the next cement block and in slow motion my body rolled to the ground.

As I fell, I remember thinking, I can redeem myself...I can get my other foot under me...this isn't happening...I will keep walking...ever in denial....ever falling to the ground. Not wanting to fall on my hands and hurt my old injuries in my wrists, I rolled my arm under my body and landed on my shoulder. Just as I landed my head hit the ground and split open my eyebrow.

Everyone there saw it. Equally, we all felt it was in slow motion and with each passing nanosecond, it looked as though I would follow through with my opposite foot and catch myself. But that is not the way it went down. Not the way I went down.

COVID...seems to be a lot like that fall.

We watched it slowly beginning. It started far, far away...first in China, the far east, then, the near east, then, Europe, and then on to the USA...we didn't think it would have much effect here. Surely, we will get our feet under us.

We're not going to fall on such a small piece of sidewalk. This part is not the roughest part we've seen before. This is too straight to trip and fall on.

In the end, I had a bleeding eyebrow, and a pulled rotator cuff.

In the end...we get dislocated.

We bleed a little, and sometimes a lot. The entire economy is bleeding and no one knows if it will coagulate? I am in denial. This can't really be happening!? I'm sure we'll be back on our feet next week.

My life turned upside down. I thought I was ready. I had made my first choice to stay at work and just not be given any hours…but, my third choice was to take a one-month leave of absence. I was sure that I could handle that. One month at home would be a nice break from the busy three months I had already worked this year.

I was not prepared for the blow to the gut when the email arrived stating that I was being laid off for 30 days, and that would be revisited, possibly be extended up to 6 months, at which time they will let me go!

Wha????? This was not what I signed up for! What do they mean, "If this goes beyond 6 months?!" The news was saying we should hit our peak mid-April… doesn't that mean we can all get back to normal by May 1? Why wouldn't we just go back to our jobs and our schools and our schedules and our vacations as soon as this is over? SIX months? This can't go on for that long! Can it?

My life changed. My secure world wasn't secure anymore. The sure footing was becoming unstable. The fall happens despite our best efforts to catch ourselves or redeem our footings.

When I fell, I lived in denial for a few days before I went to the doctor who confirmed that I had done some nasty damage to my shoulder. The eye was bruised and thankfully the bleeding had stopped. The external wound healed up a lot quicker than the internal.

Just like the fall I took on the sidewalk, this COVID-19 fall was nasty. It has done some damage. Thankfully, the bleeding isn't too bad and the CERB (Canada Emergency Response Benefit: Government assistance in Canada) has helped.

We may be a bit bruised, but those scars will heal. It's the "soft tissue" damage, internal stuff, that will take longer.

The schedules. The appointments. Doesn't even matter now if it is with the dentist or a good friend or a Bible study. Any appointment would be nice.

I haven't had a solid schedule as long as I can remember. I have always worked shift work. Now, our lives run on a schedule. We have to, otherwise the days will melt into each other and nothing will get accomplished.

Blair wakes first, and he starts his day. I get up later. By the time I get up he has already touched base with all his family who woke up 3 hours earlier than us. He has had breakfast and is watching the morning COVID-19 report.

I start a lot slower than he does, but, by 10:00 am I am busy in my sewing room, making masks for anyone and everyone. Requests come in about every other day. I don't want to commit to more than I can handle. So, far, I have made about 3 dozen.

I see Blair at lunch and head back to my sewing room. He is spending his day on the computer or the phone looking for someone, anyone who is hiring. Although he has been hired by a company, they won't do a one-on-one evaluation with him, so there is no work until he can get the proper training. So, he goes back to the phone, networking with everyone he knows.

He gets a call from time to time from the church to deliver a food basket. Every afternoon at 3:00 pm we go for a ride to join a "parade" of vehicles around the special-care home in our local area, to hold up signs and toot our horns and drive by and wave to say thank you to the nurses and workers who are fighting on the front lines.

Then, it's back sewing, or laundry, or making some dinner. Hubby knows he needs to let me do my household stuff, and not ask or expect me to watch movies or just come and go with him all day. He goes for a walk to check the mail, or for a drive, just to get out of the house.

Many times I find him standing in the window looking out at the highway behind my house. He is watching the trucks go by. I know he is crying in his heart, that THAT is what he wants to be doing. He states how this is the best time of year to be driving a truck. I have no words for him. I have nothing to comfort him with. He wants to work. He wants to provide for his family. He is doing everything possible he knows to do, and yet…it is out of his hands.

He spent the first few weeks going to bed late and getting up early. He couldn't sleep, he says. I know better; I know he's worried.

I wasn't too worried in the beginning. I was working more hours than I had this time last year. I thought I would be just fine with my job, and that would carry us through.

Blair kept saying a job for him would come next week, or by the middle of the month, or that he was certain he would be working by the following month. Each time we'd reach that time marker, the goal would be moved further away.

One day he said, "You're never gonna believe this."

Hmmm, it always makes me a bit apprehensive when he says that.

Blair told me how the peace of God just came over him that night when he went to bed. And he had the best sleep that he's had in a while. He said that he felt God was putting a knowing in his spirit that everything was going to be okay, and God had everything in His control. There was no need to worry.

That is so unlike my husband. He always wants to know where the next dollar is coming from and WHEN! Like most of us, he doesn't do well with the unknown.

What's going to happen? How long is this going to last? Will we get our jobs back when this is all over? Is this the Tribulation? Or getting ready for Armageddon?

Then, we hear other voices, like those who are saying "This is God's judgment," or "It's the government's conspiracy," and even the speculations on the news that two billion people are going to die! Where does the worry end? Will we end up in internment camps? Will it go to martial law? HAS it gone to martial law?

My mind is overwhelmed and my good friends send me posts day and night. I have to be wise and listen to what God is saying to me during this time. There are so many voices. I guess I was busy working. Thankfully, at my job I have to turn my phone off while I'm in the air. It's a nice break from all the news and noises of the world. But, now that I am not working, I am shocked at how much the TV, the phone and the computer command my time and attention.

I have had to put them down, turn them off and put them away for a portion of my day, or the burdens will be too heavy to bear.

This is a cross we all are bearing together. Yet, we are alone. When it gets right down to it. I am home…virtually alone, Although my husband is here with me, I am going through some feelings and thoughts all by myself. In the night, when I go to bed, it's just me and my soul, and God. And that's when we talk.

It's been a number of years since I remember being this raw and "real" with God. Oh, I pray, and do my "devotions" and talk to Him…but, I mean those times where I open my soul, like a torn shirt, and expose those fears I am even afraid to admit to myself. Is this the beginning of the end? This is certainly of biblical proportions.

Many a "prophetic" voice has their explanation for what is happening. Those who study the end times are piecing this into their findings. But, I'm sure the captives in WWII also thought it was the end of the world, as did many Christians throughout history.

That's why it's so important for me, now more than ever, to stay close to Jesus. When I am with Him, and I slow down enough to sit in His presence and sense He is close, my fears melt away. I wonder if this is what it was like for many saints through the ages who had to go underground, or into hiding. Seems the gospel thrives in times when life is uncertain.

I have more time for the Lord now. He is the one who is keeping me sane through all of this solitude. In the end I realize that being alone with the best Person in the universe is the best-case scenario! He is love and perfection…and perfect love casts out fear.

I don't know what tomorrow will bring, but I know Who holds tomorrow. So, Bring It On!

ABOUT THE AUTHOR

I was invited to a ladies' Bible study that met in a church gym around small tables when I met Sharon. I was new to the group and felt like a foreigner to Canada. When the leader of our table asked me to introduce myself, I talked about having a life in two places, of the dissonance and disconnect and yet the richness of belonging in both. When I was done talking, Sharon said—"I could have said every word of that—about myself. You and I are going to be friends." And we have been and I would not have missed one minute of our friendship. Sharon is one of the most giving people I know. I think we will be friends forever. Lucky me!

INTERLUDE: I WAIT

SHARON MACDONALD

in the darkness I feel all alone
In the solitude of my quiet home
I wait

in the cool of the evening
The day lights are dimming
I wait

the darkness comes in like a veil
Suddenly the world is still
I wait

like an expectant mother
Craving the dawn like no other
I wait

in peace I know will come the morning
As will leave the mourning
I wait

by labor and birth will come the new day
With revelation it's on its way

I wait

till HE calms my heart and holds my hand
And stays with me while I stand
And wait

till the night is past
It's day at last
I wait only on the Lord!

SURROUNDED BY MERCY

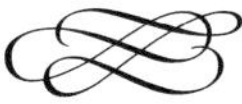

MICHELLE P.

It is dusk. The time mosquitos start biting. The time of day when the whole village smiles as the sun goes down. The time you feel you can breathe again after the suffocating heat of the day. A motorbike drives past with a carpenter and his bookshelf—off for delivery. The call to prayer gathers people from their showers, their labors, their cooking, their tea and for a moment all is still, as they engage in their evening prayers.

As the sky darkens, we begin the 30-minute process of setting up our beds under the tent in our front yard. Bamboo bases, pillows, mattresses, mosquito nets, water bottles, sheets, a torch, itch-cream, nappies and wipes, a Bible and the baby cot all make their way one by one under the shelter. Mosquitos bite us as we assemble our nighttime "camp" where it will be cooler than sleeping inside the house.

A mud-brick wall about waist height is all that is between us and our neighbors who are setting up their beds at the same time. Goats jump to and fro looking for whatever nourishment they can find in our desert land.

On this particular night, the desert seemed oppressive and exhausting. This was a normal feeling, but on this night, it was intensified. I fell asleep quickly after feeding the baby one last time and praying with my husband as was our routine. Every night we went to sleep we knew we were hidden in the crevices of God's hands, given that we were so vulnerable and a prime target for terrorism which was visibly growing in our region.

At 2 am I woke up suddenly. I was unsettled in my spirit and gripped with fear. Thoughts of harm coming to us. I checked that the children were still sleeping and lay back down on my pillow. How could I sleep under such circumstances?

The heat. The wind. The neighbors looking over the wall. The noise of the animals. The threats of violence with no barrier of a gate or lock to protect us. I sat up again.

Suddenly I saw a bright light at one corner of our tent. With a flash this light encircled our tent, drawing a line in the sand around its four corners. From this boundary line, light shot out away from the tent as if it was a shooting star.

I sat in silence and in shock. I had just seen the evidence of God's encircling presence with my own eyes. I lay back down and fell back asleep peacefully and in wonder.

That morning at breakfast we read Psalm 3: 3-6 "For you are a shield around me, O Lord. To the Lord I cry and He answers me from His holy hill. I lie down and sleep; I wake up again because the Lord sustains me. I will not fear the tens of thousands drawn up against me on every side."

We found out later that morning that travelling terrorists had spent that night a stone's throw away from our tent…peacefully causing no harm.

He truly is the One who is always watching, always attentive, and always sustaining those He loves.

ABOUT THE AUTHOR

I first met Michelle through a Facebook group of moms living in tough places—desert locations. Her insights and words and photos were all striking. She introduced me to the writings and paintings of Lilias Trotter and gave me current insights into how Lilias thoughtfully lived in North Africa over a century ago. If you have never read Lilias Trotter, this is a gem you want to find! When I met Michelle in person, she lived up to the beautiful person I had encountered on Facebook. I have gained so much by having her friendship along my journey.

INTERLUDE: A MIRROR IN THE DARKNESS

ELLEN JANZEN

One of the problems with being in isolation or suspended from life as we have commonly filled it—with lots and lots of activities, some of them purposeful distractions—is that you might find your flaws quite annoying. To yourself.

Sometimes when all your props are removed…when all you have is your raw self, you don't really like what you see. The mirror of a quiet life is not always kind to our flaws.

When a global pandemic was announced, it felt like the world started to tip on its side. The sense of sliding off the lower edge, brought up a lot of anxiety and futility—the inability to control or compensate for what was going on. Most of us got a chance to face our own inner darkness, the less attractive side of ourselves.

None of us like our dark side—we generally have enough coping energy to get past our own darkness at least a little bit. Some of us have learned to stop and take it in from time to time and process the "stuff" we've hidden away in deep caves. It isn't an easy task to do that.

When we hide things from ourselves, it's usually because it's too painful or too scary to deal with at the time.

Now in the upheaval those storage units may emerge and the emotions that surface with them are uncomfortable. Those emotions may feel overwhelming and too big to bear. Or they may feel scary or unattractive.

If that is what is happening, it is not unique to you. Many of us are facing similar "upset." We have the option and opportunity to invite Jesus to meet us in that valley. Or garbage pit—as it sometimes feels like we've unearthed decomposing matter.

There was a woman in the gospel stories who had a lot of her own shame and junk she was hiding from. She went to get water when no one else would be at the well, only to find herself in the company of a man who apparently "knew everything she ever did"—her words. Much as Jesus showed up at the well to meet the woman who didn't want to be seen—He has that same capacity to show up for you. With perfect timing.

The things you have turned away from are visible to His eye and he welcomes us to talk to him about them, even in the stages of reflection where they still are not quite clear yet. The conversation may help bring the clarity you are hoping for. Or the healing.

This is why journaling is helpful to many people. Bring some of your thoughts up from the pit of your stomach—notice where in your body you feel the frustration or the anxiety. Let the feelings be real. Give words to the physical and then search for the feeling words that seem to match.

As we look back through our memories, it's possible to recall times we felt this way before—what is the pattern of relationships that this is helping us understand?

If you can't quite remember why this feeling got to be a part of your way of facing life, ask Jesus if there is some place in your past that He wants to show you—a memory of a time when you had a similar encounter with futility or fear. And ask Him to show you what His perspective is on that time, or event, or relationship. Ask Him to be a participant in the memory and show you or speak to you about His presence.

I don't expect this to be easy when I do it, because it often entails getting in touch with my inner pain. I think of it as a tunnel I will have to walk through—to the other side of the issue. Or to another part of the journey.

John O'Donohue describes this as "suffering"—the cleansing work of getting in touch with our inner pain so that it can be brought into the light and into a place of "healing"—or redemption. Healing doesn't mean all the pain will dissipate, but it does involve the work of embracing it as part of who we are. Making room for sadness over what went wrong allows us to receive the grace to let go of the injustice or "wrong" part of what happened.

Sadness, grief and the tears that come with it—these are a gift that integrates what we wish for and what we actually have. When we allow tears to wash through us, there is a new pathway made clear, where things we experienced become a part of the wisdom we live by. Wisdom, compassion and concern for the greater good of the human community that inhabit this planet.

We will still remember the pain, but in a way that gives us freedom to live outside of it. With healing that gives us the gift of redemption that is the promise of our faith. Jesus, the redeemer.

Jesus, the one who looks on our pain with compassion. He bears our sorrows. He looks on our failings with grace. And hopes we will stop long enough to see love shining from His eyes. In our direction.

Sometimes it takes a good bout of isolation—the suspension of life's many commitments or distractions—so that we can put our energy into this inner work.

So, in some ways, for some of us, the gift of the pandemic is this nudge toward the mirror that shows us our own dark shadows. When we stop avoiding our own darkness, we often discover that Jesus, alive within us, is a brighter light giver than we ever imagined.

MY FATHER KNOWS

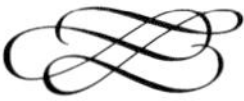

MICHELLE H.

Note from Ellen:

Because this submission comes from a personal journal entry, I've prefaced it with an introduction to Michelle's circumstances.

Widowed April 7, 2019, Michelle lost more than her best friend and husband. She also lost her work supporting his ministry, their home in North Africa, and her many precious relationships there. She found herself relocating to the USA and suddenly a single parent to their autistic adolescent child, who needed 24/7 supervision and was terrified to engage in even simple everyday outings like going to grocery stores or church. Because he could not be left alone and could not overcome his fear of going out, Michelle also lost her liberty and the opportunity to focus on her own needs to grieve while she spent months not leaving her home, seeking to go through the paperwork and applications required by agencies that might give her caregiving assistance and respite care. When COVID-19 forced the world into lockdown in the spring of 2020, life for the two of them changed very little. Its primary effect was to further delay Michelle's application processes, increasing the pressure on her to carry on for many more months of 24/7 caregiving with no respite. Yet, it is clear from her journal entries during the spring of 2020 that the Lord worked in Michelle's heart during this season, helping her grieve loss and turn her focus toward Himself—the Source of all strength and hope.

April 7 - a day forever etched deeply into my mind and heart. Last evening, I remembered the dream I had last year on this night. In my dream, I had witnessed

Mark disappearing from his hospital room, accompanied by the angel I called "Lightsaber Guy." I remembered the powerful joy my heart felt for Mark while I was dreaming. A few minutes later, there was a knock on my door and I got confirmation - it was not just a dream. Mark was gone. He went home.

I realized that I wanted a way to spend some time today celebrating resurrection, doing an activity that causes me to feel joy. And it hit me—I could make paper flowers. That craft had delighted my heart last week. So, I started a bouquet of Easter lilies.

They aren't done yet, but what fun! As I sat cutting and folding and gluing in the living room while my son and I watched the movie "Sing," I felt light and free. I was playing. I thought, "Hey, this is something I could do every year if I wanted—a new tradition!" Each step in making the blooms was a new way to worship.

Later this evening, my adult daughter and her husband plan to come over to stand distant from us on the front lawn and remember together. Remember Daddy, remember the love for him that will always be in our hearts, and remember that our home is heaven.

John 11:25 NLT

Jesus told her, 'I am the resurrection and the life. Anyone who believes in me will live, even after dying.'

The detail about Easter that has stood out to me this year is the forgiveness, love, and power of Jesus as he was dying. I read a commentary about Luke 23[1] and a few concepts jumped from the page…

Remember James and John asking to be given the honor of sitting at Jesus' right and left when he sits on His throne? Jesus said they had no idea what they were asking, spoke of it involving huge suffering, and said the Father would put those He chose into those positions.

Fast forward. There He is, in His crown of thorns with a sign declaring His identity as King and He is hanging between two thieves, the ones chosen by the Father for that honor, on His right and on His left.

One of the thieves threw insults when Jesus forgave their crucifiers. The other was repentant. He asked to be remembered when Jesus came into His kingdom. Jesus' words to him have been ringing in my mind a lot this week, "I promise you that today you will be with Me in Paradise."

Today—it is immediate somehow, this life in the eternal realm. It makes me see dying like a doorway.

Paradise—a beautiful, secure, Kingly garden, a place of rest. I think MacLaren got it right when he said: "'With me' makes 'Paradise' wherever a soul is."

MacLaren wrote that although Jesus was taunted that He must be powerless, "His refusal to use His power to save Himself proved Him the Son of God." He was there to pay the price of sin for all humanity in all of time—including the soldiers and rulers and thief who mocked him. And He, the Resurrection and the Life, died physically to make a way for the penitent thief and all who believe to have life and rest with Him.

Then, Sunday, He rose physically, too!! Death is defeated! Joy!!

It is different somehow, for me now, thinking about the empty tomb. I always thought of it as victorious and powerful, but now the hope it gives touches my heart with shocking joy! My companion and best friend, Mark, on loan to me for the last 32 years, is now—wow!—hanging out in that garden with the King!

These last couple of days have had some challenges and tears, yet victories, too. Easter Sunday morning my son and I joined the livestream morning worship service, then watched the last hour of the Gospel of John movie, then sang together again many Easter favorites.

In the late afternoon Easter Day, I felt a deep sadness as I walked outside around the house. Once again, my son had refused to leave the house, afraid that Coronavirus would be in the air. He lifted weights and danced inside the house while I walked in circles around the house, wept, and prayed. I told the Lord how much I miss my life. He met with me in such a special way as I poured out to Him my aching loss!

My friend named this experience, as I described it to her, lamenting. Yeah. That is what it is. And I sensed, without really knowing why, that it was important. It was healing, somehow, to bring my losses into the light and speak them in God's presence. I named them and acknowledged out loud why each one hurt. As I did, I humbled my heart before Him. He knows, knew beforehand, the violation and mutilation my soul would feel. His grace is so amazing! He heard and saw my raw emotions and His love settled over each one.

My African friend, Kimi, sent these words to me—an anonymous hymn…

He knows the bitter, weary way,
The endless striving day by day,
The souls that weep, the souls that pray—
My Father knows,
My Father knows.

He knows how hard the fight has been,
The clouds that come our lives between,
The wounds the world has never seen—
My Father knows,
My Father knows.

He knows, when faint and worn we shrink,
How deep the pain, how near the brink,
Of dark despair we pause and shrink—
My Father knows,
My Father knows.

Isa 57:15

For this is what the high and exalted One says—he who lives forever, whose name is holy:
"I live in a high and holy place, but also with the one who is contrite and lowly in spirit, to
revive the spirit of the lowly and to revive the heart of the contrite.

---

1. Alexander MacLaren, *MacLaren's Commentary: Expositions of Holy Scripture*, Harrington, DE: DelMarva Publications, 2013.

INTERLUDE: A SPRINKLE OF LOVE

ELLEN JANZEN

The sun has kissed my face
and left its prints
across my nose.

I was unhurried in the garden
chasing a dragonfly
and dodging mosquitoes.

There was water to deliver
to a drooping plant
and worms to watch;

I lost track of the daylight —
Sunshine above my head.

When I came in
there was a rosy glow
that had not been there
when I started.

The marks of love
of unremitting warmth

and the promise of tomorrow…
run like a line of disorderly ants
across my nose
where the sun has freckled me
with a sprinkling of kisses.

FROM A ROOM WITHOUT A VIEW

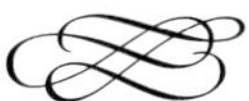

ELLEN JANZEN

Tonight could be another sleepless night, with my thoughts out in the wind at the base of the mountains where I live. There is rain on my roof, a sound I love. But I don't think it will be enough to lull me to sleep.

There are too many things that I have managed to not think about all day. I will lie here with my thoughts, wishing for sleep. Waiting.

The first time I struggled to get to sleep was in boarding school. Sleep was not an enemy until I was alone in my bed in the dorm room I shared with someone who wasn't part of my family. I found it hard to sleep, night after night.

I was five years old when I first started to make my own bed, changing my sheets on Monday after school. Each dorm had a designated day to strip their beds and get clean sheets. Life was governed by schedules, not love. I turned six without fanfare in the stark contours of dorm life.

I survived well. I was cute and funny and smart enough in school—I rarely got punished. My struggle was private—it was the fear that came between getting into bed and finding sleep in the dark after hard days of fending for myself.

I could handle the loneliness of daylight hours—but night was a different story. I learned to bury some of my fears and all of my pains. If the day had been hard, I didn't tell anyone. But I skirted the edge of sleep for as long as I could, avoiding the dreams that I knew might come.

The next year my parents moved to the city and I lived at home again. I have no memory of any difficulty falling asleep for the next few years. In fact, my memories of that time are like an orange grove—sun-kissed. A season of sweet fruit. Sadly, one that didn't last longer.

Seven years after boarding school days my sleepless nights returned to harass me. Once again, I faced down the darkest of nights—outside and deep inside me. I would lie in bed where we still lived in the city—not in a dorm in a country school. A few blocks away the city clock chimed each quarter hour and I would count the bells as I snuffed out any pain within.

My mom had died in the first weeks of my seventh year in school. She had been ill for the holidays and now she was gone, and a gigantic wave of pain threatened to engulf my life and disintegrate me in its swell. But I evaded that pain, as I had those many years ago. Perhaps my skills from boarding school gave me the edge I needed to get through each day.

Still, each night, I was at the mercy of the clock tower. Sleep was not my friend.

I learned to endure the cycle yet again—alone. I couldn't bear the pain of longing for my mom to come to comfort me in the wounding of her absence. I buried all my feelings as deeply as I could. As well as any child is able to do. My dark cavern of grief was deep.

Eventually I found a way to live with the storm inside.

Until it was too much.

And eventually it was too much. The futility of the losses piled up and created a volcano that burst through me. If you haven't experienced childhood loss you probably would conclude I had no self control. It looked like rage. But I had held on to too much for too long and it was the grief that finally ripped me apart.

Twenty years later, I lived in a city where I had no friends who spoke my language, where conversations were about vegetables and cake and who was doing what in school. In that kind of isolation, I lost my power of reserve and the cave crashed inward on my soul. And I knew that the anger was really grief, or at least I finally figured it out.

I began to let the sorrow out, one tear at a time. At least at first. And then in rivers.

During a year when tears were beginning to cascade with a life force of their own, a friend invited me to a silent retreat. In the middle of an otherwise uneventful summer, she asked if I would like to come to Vancouver Island and spend a week with ten women in a monastery on the edge of a lake. She would cover the cost—a gift.

I had wanted to experience a silent retreat for some time, having read about them and having turned to the mysterious gift of prayer in the isolation of living in a desert country—I yearned for the richness I had heard about in long silent spaces. Days spent in a space shared only with God.

The idea of being alone and silent in a house of worship tempted the curiosity in me. It didn't occur to me to be nervous or afraid.

I had sat for seven hours on numerous occasions among a group of women whose language I only understood if they slowed down to talk to me as if I were my eight-year-old daughter. I could follow what they said to her, but in an adult conversation I was lost.

Silence had become a comfortable friend.

My week at the island monastery was a gentle gift. On the first day, as I lay on the bed with the fan blowing across the room, I looked at myself to make sure I was still physically present. The air from the fan felt like it was blowing right through me—carrying me away to another place. A place of deep rest.

My friend had told me about a tiny chapel in the basement of the main house. Some people called it The Womb, she said. It was available for anyone to use—a space to sit and pray or listen or contemplate. She predicted that amazing things could happen in there, that the sense of being enclosed took you to a different expression of trust and faith.

The room was just big enough for a bench on each side and an altar at the end with a cross on it. As I closed the door, the cross would disappear and there I would sit. Just sit. With the door closed it was pitch black inside. By design or not, it was an encased space—like a womb, as she had described. Silent. Dark. Full of rest.

I found myself there every day, some time before the dinner hour. If I didn't stay for long enough, for fear that someone else might be waiting, I would come back later. I noticed it was rarely occupied so I stayed longer and longer each day. The comfort of this room seemed to beckon me away from the walking trail through beautiful trees around the lake—something I also enjoyed. But this room went beyond the ordinary experiences of silence.

It was like a hug from the past. A return to a time when I was never alone, never forgotten, hidden deep inside my mother—the answer to her prayers. A treasured child she carried within.

And I started to heal. In the black depths of that tiny chapel the darkness of my inner cave found a way to seep out. Not in tears or in anguish but in a quiet acknowledgement that I was full of the weight of a buried grief. A thousand unshed tears stored up in my soul, waiting for the dark of night to be released. Needing this space to find my own inner labyrinth of both sadness and the gift of remembering—I was a treasure.

And finally, also, the added gift of being able to let go of the anger.

Anger not at the loss of my mother, but at the ways my stepmother had displaced her. Exquisitely embroidered lace curtains were pronounced "boring," taken down and replaced with garish orange polyester. Photos were disposed of, dishes were declared ugly. And of course our house was remade into a home for my dad's new wife.

I could see my stepmother needed to make the house into her own home, but she did so without any effort to care for our wounds or acknowledge our losses. And some of those changes were far too personal. Too personal to tell anyone how deeply they shamed me.

Here in this womb-chapel I saw my hidden pain surface and the wax that encased my heart melting, slowly, to release the bitterness of my anger. And finally, I felt invited to release myself by offering forgiveness to my stepmother. Forgiveness I would never speak of with her—she never realized how much damage she had done, so I alone benefited from that gift of letting go.

But it took a week without words and a room without a view—a time of removing all the distractions and activities of life. It was also the removal of all the words that could try to explain the sorrow that surfaced—words failed to express this deep need. It took silence and trust and darkness and perhaps this was linked to the time when I was protected in my mom's womb. Perhaps in that pre-birth memory of being fully safe, I could open my heart and let the sorrow and anger rise up to meet with mercy and grace.

In that week of choosing to be alone with God I found a place, a tiny dark chapel that made it possible for me to open the deep doors that had held my life together for far too long.

INTERLUDE: THE GOOD LUCK MUG

SARAH BAHIRAEI

If you ever come to our home, you'll probably be greeted with a cup of tea no matter the season. Admittedly, not by me—I'm still learning the art of tea-making —but by my husband. And don't expect the instant tea-bag-dunked-in-hot-water kind. No, you will be given slowed-brewed Persian chai—black tea leaves with hints of cinnamon and cardamom, steeped all morning over a low open flame on the stove.

And there might be a chance you'll reach into the kitchen cabinet for a glass and unknowingly grab the red mug. It's a small, stout ceramic cup, half-submerged in vermillion red paint, half left as natural clay. We have a green and blue one too.

They're handmade by a Turkish potter, getting his clay from the river running through our town, spinning them on his wheel and firing them in his kiln down the street.

But the red mug? That's our good luck mug.

It's called that not because it mystically brings years of good fortune and success to the drinker (at least not that we know of). It's not because it's pretty and unique— and it is, made locally and one-of-a-kind. There isn't one like it. Even its siblings who sit quietly in a row on the store shelf all look slightly different from each other upon closer inspection.

It's called our good luck mug because it has cracks—actually, a lot of cracks. Actually, the handle has been broken off and glued back together three different times in four different places. There are thick clumps of dried superglue oozing out of the broken areas and little paint chips sprinkled around the rim. 'Good luck' in a tongue-in-cheek sort of way because the glued-on handle has, on more than one occasion, slowly and melodramatically separated from the rest of the mug while in use.

Life holds a lot of cracks, doesn't it?

Our miserable-looking mug, in all its fractures and pitiful glue attempts, brings to mind the stories of grief we all carry, how life has the power to crack us wide open. I have yet to meet someone who isn't shouldering a rucksack of grief—past or present, big or small, seen or hidden. At the moment, we are all living in the same state of cracks as we experience a global pandemic, and with that brings in worry for high-risk loved ones, disappointment from canceled plans, and the loss of any sense of normalcy.

My husband and I have experienced ongoing grief before; this feeling isn't new to us. It wasn't just one defining moment or one break down the middle, but a series of blows and burials of dreams. We haven't seen much come to fruition, or at least not many prayers answered in ways we had hoped. Any appearance of control we thought we possessed has been jostled out of our hands. Add on to that a pandemic, living in a foreign country, and the upcoming birth of our first child and our stress has been turned up one too many notches.

On a macro-level, we are all enduring the world turning upside down. And with that, there's been a lot of online content lately written by well-meaning people who are trying to be encouraging during this time of heightened uncertainty. In a benevolent effort to ease the discomfort of quarantine and social distancing, there has been a flood of to-do lists, checklists, advice, and examples of productive routines infiltrating our inboxes. Get up early, exercise every day, bake bread, organize the junk drawer, write letters, Zoom in meetings, get creative, be grateful, find a new normal.

But coming from someone who has had prolonged uncertainty as a constant sidekick for the past three years, let me be the first to tell you that you don't have to do any of that. It's too much pressure when the world feels a little too shaky. When tomorrow is shadowed in the unknown, sometimes we need to survive before we think about thriving. Often, it is more essential to acknowledge how we feel for a little while before we choose all the "shoulds" thrown our way.

This grief—a crack on the handle here, a chip around the rim there—can teach us the importance of holding space. In her book, *The Broken Way*, Ann Voskamp suggests, "Maybe wholeness is embracing brokenness as part of your life."[1] And when life throws a curveball, like an outbreak of a novel virus, we hold on to hope, which cannot be held on to without a few cracks. Grief, cracks, wholeness, and hope. They're the ingredients to a recipe for fertile and holy ground. Welcome it.

If your good luck mug has cracks like mine—perhaps from the strange state of the world or from something else entirely—hold space for it. Don't take sandpaper to it and buff out the discomfort by way of routines and productivity just yet. Identify the grief you're feeling. Look for the growth among the cracks. Doing so can make way for wholeness. Joy and grief can be felt simultaneously. Imperfections and beauty can live side-by-side. And know this: the cracks are not fragile despite their appearance. They are being held together tightly by the Potter, the one who created the mug, the one who sees, who resurrects, who makes all things new.

When life feels unresolved and the threads of simply being are left untied, come to our house—you'll be in like-minded company. Pull up the comfy chair, the one over there in the corner with the throw pillows. We'll offer you that good, Middle Eastern chai. Choose the ramshackle cup with the crimson red paint and embrace both the defects and beauty. Hold space for grief in this time of uncertainty. Trust that the cracks will lead to light.

And, while I cannot prove this for sure, I'm almost certain everything tastes just a little bit better and a little bit sweeter in that good luck mug.

This was first published in Sarah's blog onefootonboth.com

---

1. Ann Voskamp, *The Broken Way: A Daring Path into the Abundant Life*, Grand Rapids, MI: Zondervan, 2016.

WILD DONKEY WANDERING

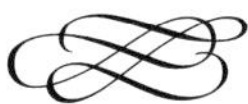

HOPE HESSED

Ok, friends O'Mine, forgive me this but know from the get-go there's something about donkeys that I've always loved and admired. However, around the world they've gotten a loser reputation. BUT I think it's mostly undeserved.

My family went to the Grand Canyon when I was 7, and what was the one souvenir I wanted? A little donkey. Maybe God does indeed start speaking to us much, much younger than we imagine.

Anyway, here's a bit of proof to back up my claim that these maligned animals are admirable. First of all, Balaam's donkey is the only recorded animal to speak (other than that snake). He didn't only speak but also saw an angel and passed on a message. And the kicker for us: Jesus chose to come on a donkey—even the foal of a donkey—when he was lauded as king. What kind of a crazy honor is that for a baby donkey? I wonder what the rest of that donkey baby's life was like…

So, all that to say please don't get insulted when I compare you/us to donkeys… Come on, you know as well as I do, if you are honest…we're all jack*sses sometimes.

But redeemed s-s-sinners we are—made to carry the glory of our LORD.

As I look back over life from the vantage of 6 decades (that sounds so much better than the actual number) I wonder. As an always-single Christ-follower (in America for the first 40 and the last 20 in a Muslim country), during the many seasons of aloneness/isolation that fill life, I've discovered some of these seasons have been emotional, some spiritual AND emotional, and some physical. These times are never fun. Rather, they are dry, desert-dwelling times.

For many years I've seen myself as a plodder. The only verse I memorized in high school and still know including its address is *1 Corinthians 15:58*:

> *Therefore my beloved brethen*
> *Be steadfast*
> (plod on)
> *Immovable*
> (stay in the race God has marked out for you)
> *Always abounding in the work of the Lord*
> (plod plod plod…do the next right thing)
> *Knowing your toil*
> (keep pulling that plow one slow step at a time)
> *Is not in vain*
> (all you/we donkeys do is pull the plow (never alone) but someone
>   else plants the seeds).

And so, I've plodded on, making these the goals of my life, no matter where I am.

There are not a lot of actual things I know how to do. I can't sing well or play an instrument. I can't do mechanical things, plumb, sledge or connect electrical wires. These are all things that would be extremely useful in this life where I've found myself.

However, I am well equipped for plodding and steadfastness. Maybe more so

because I've watched my mom be steadfast when she felt alone as a navy wife— wait that's another story…one for her to tell.

When I think of plodding and being steadfast (another way to say sure-footed, just like those Grand Canyon donkeys!), it's these steady animals that come to mind.

So, this is what I've aspired to be.

Steady and immovable—yes, like a donkey.

———————

Yet, many times I've found myself feeling more like

"Wild Donkey Wandering Alone."

The wilderness/desert-isolation times are like this. I find myself biting (or at least trying to), kicking, putting myself on display heehawing and trampling good gardens in my dissatisfaction.

These times of isolation have included:

-Being single in my 30s and 40s and beyond, in American evangelical churches. Singleness is often not regarded as a plausible godly best in my experience. Therefore, many young Christ following women feel isolated and as if something is wrong with them. Many have wondered when, if, and why God has not given them the gifts of the promised man, whoops I mean promised land. Thus, dwelling too long in

The Land of Why Not?

-Not having the "ambition" to climb the prescribed Western ladder of success. Therefore, I've experienced mocking and being looked down on as if I'm not "adult" enough or good enough somehow. Oh, what wild donkey kicking havoc this can wreak in one's soul.

The Land of Not Enough.

-Living in a very foreign culture without enough language to understand what's going on around me much of the time. Added to this, the assumption by most Westerners that simply because I've lived there for many years, I am fluent—this assumption and the guilt I've heaped on myself, expectations of my own reinforced by others, causes great aloneness. I believe dwelling in

The Land of Expectations and Comparisons

is one of the greatest desert/isolation quicksands we can land in.

-Being in the country of my birth with no landing spot, along with few people who understand this is no longer "home." After a few years I realized I no longer really belong in either place. Forgetting how to say things in my native tongue, or how to turn on a television, have a way of making you feel like you are in

The Land of Not Belonging.

-Experiencing the greatest grief of my life, the sudden physical death of my dearest 11-year-old boy. Too distraught and confused to care about being sensitive to cultural norms, too sad and stunned to even bite and kick (at least for the first few months). Mostly just wildly wondering and wandering in

The Land of What Is Happening?!!!!!

Wild Donkey Wandering Indeed.

———————————

It is only after much lashing out according to my wild donkey ways, when I can do nothing but crumple, after self-pity then comes dark, dark sadness. When I can finally speak my aloneness, sadness, desperate-not-good-enough-ness, then, I can hear…

or not.

Sometimes in these times God is silent and/or completely hidden from my eyes, ears, and touch. In these desert days when guilt and the fiery farts (lots of lies and hot air in these) of Satan tempt me to despair, all I can do is sob, and look upward. Often the clouds are so thick and dark (literally, emotionally, and spiritually) all I can do is muster a teeny bit of hope reminding myself the Sun/Son is up there somewhere…

These days often stay dark so all I can do is plod 1 or 2 steps. In these most dreary silent days, I can only do the ONE next thing. The one next thing may be: read to a kiddo, do the dishes, sit with people silently because there are NO words, yet loving them with my presence OR simply murmuring:

Jesus have mercy on us

Jesus have mercy on us

Over and over.

Other days when I'm so angry (again) I can only walk and rage, trying to hear words of grace and hope in music, the sounds of nature, or giggling children. The voice of God does resound in unexpected ways when one listens. Even donkeys making their truly indescribable noises as well as birds can speak of God's attention to us. Listening and watching the clear communication of the same birds that fascinated my sweet boy, remind me that they are perhaps messengers between earth and paradise.

Birds also remind me that my anchor is attached to the Throne of God Above. The anchor chain comes down, wraps around me and holds me secure. This image has sustained me and reassured me when I cannot see The Hidden Face of God.[1] I realize even in my raging:

O God where else do I have to go? I will not walk away.

The burning bush from which Moses heard God's voice was off the beaten path. He saw it and then he had to go over to it…and take off his shoes. I'm convinced there are times when I've seen or heard a bush burning and I refused to go and look and listen. A nudging of the Spirit and yet I chose to look away or make myself busy (Facebook, TV, food, spending, and so on) when I knew I should/could investigate the nudge. Instead, I often walk into my self-sorryness. I go to the deep Sahara of self-sorryness or even back to the self-sorryness of slavery that this desert dwelling time is leading me out of. This self-sorryness scars so many others around me as I lash out…

YET it takes not even a step but a pivot to begin. A slight turning can become a full pivot eventually. A look choosing to face the Sun-Son even when it's too cloudy or dark to see. A turn, a confession cry of "Help me in my UNBELIEF," is the beginning. At times we need Jesus' physical hands as well…although they are not always available to us in the dark desert. Yet they and He will come. Usually not in the way we expect or want. We most likely have to open our eyes, ears, and hands, maybe even our nose, but these are the times we need to ask others to hold up our arms so we can learn again to feel God's presence come down.

My arm holders are almost always physically far from me. I hate that and wish it were not the case. But the fact is: in this broken, less than ideal world, we are broken and often physically separated and feel alone. The fact is:

He will never leave us alone.

We, as Christ followers, have to live in

The Land of Paradoxes and Conundrums

We feel alone, YET in fact we are NOT.

Jesus is KING, YET His royal entry was made as a baby and then He came in power on the foal of a donkey.

We are broken, YET not shaken.

We are dust, YET we have HIS power available to us.

The list goes on and on…. Learning to embrace these as well as Jesus' no-s helps me get back on course. This is so easy to say and so hard to do! Making Grateful

Lists each day, even of teeny tiny things, can jump start your turning back. Admitting brokenness, living honestly, crying out for help in our unbelief, for help period...these are the humble beginnings of a path out of desert dwelling.

But make no mistake—because we are broken, we will have times in the desert. We are human and we FORGET TO REMEMBER. It is in the desert of aloneness and suffering we become more real, more intimate, more aware of His kindness and tender mercies, His inexpressible Hesed.[2]

Asking God to enable me to see this world from a heavenly perspective rather than only an earthly one has been life settling for me. These Holy Spirit-given glimpses are the gifts by which he has settled my wild wandering donkey self. From wilderness wandering to a usable, yoked with Jesus, plowing steadfast plodder, immovable, abounding in the work of the Lord...knowing my toil is not in vain.

Someday instead of wild donkeys wandering alone,
When we live fully in the light of the Sun of Righteousness
And revere His Name
We will instead be:
Spring calves set free from the stall —
Kicking and jumping for JOY.

HOW TO CULTIVATE REMEMBERING:

Tell each other what He has done.

Listen to others.

Write down what He's doing.

Know the stories of how He's worked in the past.

Bow before Him alone and together.

Look for His daily kindness.

Imitate His daily kindness.

It's His kindness that Leads us to repentance.

YET will I trust His Unfailing LOVE.

---

1. *The Hidden Face of God* is the title of an album and book by Michael Card that has much influenced my wanderings of the past 3 grief-stricken years of my life. Michael Card, *The Hidden Face of God: Finding the Missing Door to the Father Through Lament*, Carol Stream, IL, Tyndale, 2014.
2. *Inexpressible* is the title of a book by Michael Card that has put words to God's tenderness to me in this most recent period of global isolation. Michael Card, *Inexpressible: Hesed and the Mystery of God's Lovingkindness*, Downers Grove, IL, IVP Books, 2018.

ABOUT THE AUTHOR

We've come to the last of my friends, but certainly, by no means is Hope the least. She is perhaps one of my most unique friends, going places and being part of a community in a way that is rare and very precious. And, as a result, she has paid a high cost in suffering. It has been one of the deepest honours of my life to walk through a dark valley with Hope and to see her lift her eyes and see the strength of the hills around her—and the "help" that comes from the Maker of those hills. I believe she would trek through mountains for her friends, on dark and stormy nights—I admire and love her for her persistence and tenacity.

INTERLUDE: EMPTY SPACE, WAITING SPACE, STILL SPACE

ELLEN JANZEN

There is a space inside of you—perhaps it is your soul…or your spirit, I am not entirely sure—but a space that is "you." No one else can get there but you. No one can describe it, no one can fill it, no one can reach it—unless you invite them.

Even God waits for an invitation. God the Spirit has the capacity to see and know you—but he waits. God: the one who designed you as a human masterpiece. God: who invented the magnificent and unique combination that make up your mind and soul…and yes, your body as well.

God is there—at your invitation, in that space that is only yours, waiting for the still moments when you might notice. God, who is life itself.

Each breath we take is a divine gift—from an infinite source of all life.

The first time I recognized this was in the still silence after a (relatively easy) home birth. I looked back and reflected on the hard work and quiet joy of bringing a child out of my body into the world. I felt the breath of God on my soul.

It was breath-taking. Sorry for the pun. I'm not trying to be funny or cheap or… anything at all, really. The glimpse of eternity took my breath away. I paused and stopped breathing for the next few seconds as I pondered deeply what I had encountered in this birth.

I gave birth four times, but never noticed my baby take their first breath—even the last one who didn't breathe without help for eight whole minutes. During those eight minutes I knew I had to give her life back to God—it felt like I faced a tiny doorway into hell. The idea of losing her. Hell, the opposite of life.

She finally breathed, starting so gradually I didn't see the transition. Her breathing was a tangle of oxygen tubes and then supported in an incubator for 4 more days. Every breath a gift. Her life a gift.

When my grandson was born, quietly and without difficulty, I finally watched a baby's first breath. It was the most magnificent thing. His silent, still chest rising with a first inhale to invite the world in.

Again:

Life is a gift.

I dare not forget it.

We are wholly dependent on God for our lives. We are only whole when we realize how deeply we need him in our inner world—when we find our connection between our finite soul and His infinite goodness and love.

God becomes part of your inner space—at your invitation. He enters and then waits for the still moments, for you to notice. The times when you are stopped and all that is going on is that you are breathing deeply of the oxygen of life. He is there as your silence turns your ears toward Him…

You will hear, or perhaps feel, the breath of God's life, in unison with your own.

But first, it is highly probable that you will feel unsettled. Being silent is not as easy as it sounds. Initially, for most of us, silence unravels a few knots we have kept tied together in secret, sometimes even a secret from ourselves.

Often, we have a rush of thoughts or a physical reaction to the silence and aloneness that we feel. For me this often happens in the pit of my stomach, a feeling of turmoil tumbles like a washing machine as buried emotions rise from deep within me. I get to choose to pay attention to these deep secrets that are surfacing—or not. If it is too much all at once, sometimes I need to look away.

But I don't stay away.

I come back to silence and enter the relationship with my deeper self again, paying attention to what my "gut" is telling or releasing in me. I get as still as I am able. Come back to focus each time my mind wanders.

Eventually the silence starts to feel familiar and I find more than my own thoughts there. I sense God-my-Creator as a present companion.

The beauty of connection to the sovereign, all-loving Creator will stop you. It will stop your automatic in and out breathing. Even just for a few seconds. And it will give you a new perspective, a new way to see. A new appreciation for the powerful Love that runs the universe.

Psalm 46:10 says,

Be still and know that I am God.

If you can take in that the one who made you is smiling into your moment of awareness, it will change who you are and who you are becoming. It may take you months of challenging practice to feel like you have found that stillness. You might have to confront a myriad of worries or distractions before you get to stillness.

But the promise is there. You will find God. Here within you—at your invitation. Above all things, He is patient and faithful and will wait while you wade through the noise to get to the silence.

A practical suggestion for this? Find a park bench, or better yet, set one up in your back yard, or on your deck, or in your kitchen if you have to. And sit for a while.

Learn to breathe slowly and let go of some of the thoughts that push you toward always getting something done. Let go of some worries and frustrations—tears might help. And just sit in the waiting place. Like a yearning mother or a greying grandpa or a doting auntie holding a sleeping child. Sit in the softness of the moment.

Learn to be still and wait.

Wait for as long as you have to, as often as you can. Because this business of finding God in the stillness—seeking Him in the quiet of a cave carved into ancient Rock? It's a hobby…a habit…an addiction for some of us—you'll see for yourself if you do this.

This flavour, the flavour that comes from sharing a moment of stillness with the true Lover of your soul—the One who made you, this is the beauty of the human experience, captured into your own inner space. The space that is you. The painting that expresses your unique art. Your soul.

A STORY OF YOUR OWN:

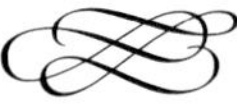

We hope you will conclude this book with a story of your own. Our gathering of stories began with this question:

When was God near to me in a hard time?

What did I gain from that?

How can we (collectively) look forward, through this misty fog we are in and remember that time and know that God will be faithful in the days to come?

Tell your story to yourself—draw it, write it, sing it…dance it—

And you can send it to me[1] if you are willing.

But listen to what the Spirit is saying to you through the lens of God's faithfulness in your own life. And be curious and courageous as you step into this day.

---

1. You can write to me at ellen@ellenjanzen.com.

THIS PAGE IS FOR YOU: WHAT IS YOUR
STORY?